Lifelong Health: Achieving Optimum Well-Being at Any Age

Anthony A. Goodman, M.D., F.A.C.S.

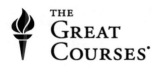

THE
GREAT
COURSES®

PUBLISHED BY:

THE GREAT COURSES
4840 Westfields Boulevard, Suite 500
Chantilly, Virginia 20151-2299
1-800-832-2412
Fax—703-378-3819
www.thegreatcourses.com

Copyright © The Teaching Company, 2010

Printed in the United States of America

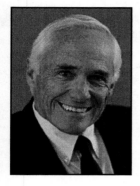

Anthony A. Goodman, M.D., F.A.C.S.

Adjunct Professor of Medicine
Montana State University

D r. Anthony A. Goodman received his B.A. from Harvard College and his M.D. from Cornell Medical College. He trained as a surgical intern and resident at the University of Michigan Medical Center in Ann Arbor and completed his surgical training and served as chief resident at the Harvard Surgical Service of Boston City Hospital, New England Deaconess Hospital, Lahey Clinic, and Cambridge City Hospital.

Dr. Goodman served as a surgeon on the hospital ship for Project HOPE and served with the U.S. Army Medical Corps from 1971 to 1973. From 1973 to 1992, he was a general surgeon, specializing in the surgical treatment of cancer, and was Clinical Associate Professor of Surgery at the University of Miami School of Medicine. In 1991, he was Visiting Professor of Surgery at the Christchurch Clinical School of Medicine in Christchurch, New Zealand.

Dr. Goodman has served as an examiner for the American Board of Surgery. He is a Fellow of the American College of Surgeons and a Diplomate of the American Board of Surgery. He has been a member of the American Society of Colon and Rectal Surgeons and the British Association of Surgical Oncology. He was the founder of the Broward Surgical Society. He has published numerous papers on both clinical and experimental surgery.

At present, Dr. Goodman is Adjunct Professor of Medicine in the WWAMI Medical Sciences Program at Montana State University, where he teaches gross anatomy, and Affiliate Professor in the Department of Biological Structure at the University of Washington School of Medicine.

Dr. Goodman is also the author of a work of historical fiction, *The Shadow of God: A Novel of War and Faith* (Sourcebooks Landmark, 2002). ■

Acknowledgments

In the preparation of this lecture series, I was fortunate to have the support of my medical colleagues at Montana State University, as well as friends and family members, including Troy Bertlesen, Deidre Combs, Poppy Gard, Janice Haugen, Robert Radice, and Diane Zantop. All gave generously of their time, talents, and insights in their various areas of expertise, making this a much richer and deeper course offering by far.

I especially want to acknowledge my wife, Maribeth Goodman, who collaborated with me from the beginning on course design, research, and writing. Maribeth has helped me enjoy a healthier, happier, and, I believe, longer life. My fondest wish is that this course will help you do the same.

A percentage of the professor royalties from this course will be donated to the PACE Center for Girls Teresa Haran Radice Health & Wellness Center.

Disclaimer

This series of lectures is intended to increase your knowledge of nutrition, exercise, and health-related lifestyle choices and their basic effects on the human body. They are not designed for use as medical references to diagnose, treat, or prevent medical illnesses or trauma. Neither The Teaching Company nor Dr. Anthony Goodman is responsible for your use of this educational material or its consequences. If you have questions about the diagnosis, treatment, or prevention of a medical condition or illness, you should consult your personal physician.

Table of Contents

Table of Contents

Lifelong Health:
Achieving Optimum Well-Being at Any Age

Scope:

There is a little-known aspect of human aging that few of us—including me, until recently—consider: There is no scientific or medical way to determine the age of any individual human being. People can tell us their age or show us a birth certificate, but beyond that, there is no science that can put an age or date of birth on someone. We have no annual rings, as trees do; no way to count teeth, the way we do with horses. There are no biopsies or technologies that enable us to examine DNA or tissues that would allow even the most sophisticated scientist to give us an accurate age. The most we can do is guess, generally with perhaps a 10- or 20-year range. To me, this opens a wonderful door to a hopeful future, for it allows us to aspire to a long and healthy life with few constraints as to how we might choose to live that life. The possibilities for healthy, productive, and joyful years ahead of us seem, in many ways, limitless.

What, then, can each of us do to achieve and maintain optimum health and well-being? Although conventional wisdom has shown that 35 to 40 percent of longevity might be determined by genes, 60 to 65 percent is within your control, which means that *you have a choice in how you are going to live*. My overall objective in this course is to help you see your options and make educated health-related decisions for a lifetime of good health and well-being.

In this course, we present an accessible, science-based program to help preserve your health and enhance your quality of life at any age. The lectures explain how and why the body and mind age and how you can build the pillars of a health-maintenance program: good nutrition, beneficial exercise, stress-relieving relaxing and restorative activities, and more and varied healthful lifestyle choices. We will explore and redefine the currently misunderstood concepts of those pillars of good health within the context of evidence-based medicine and anecdotal evidence. And, of course, my more than 40 years of experience in the medical profession allow me to draw some reasonable conclusions, which I will share when appropriate.

We will begin this course by studying the physiological, psychological, and cultural components of aging. In addition, we will look at general misconceptions and myths about aging, talk about ways to prevent illness and enhance good health, and investigate some of the medical advancements on the horizon. Then we will turn to the first pillar of our health maintenance program: nutrition. In the nutrition lectures, I will emphasize the idea that "diet" should be defined as "a way of eating" as opposed to "a way to lose weight." We will focus on

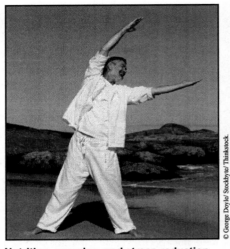

Nutrition, exercise, and stress reduction are the pillars of a healthy lifestyle.

eating healthy, fresh, whole foods; explore a wide array of alternatives to some of today's popular rigid diet programs; and learn practical eating habits that will serve us for a lifetime.

In our lectures about beneficial exercise, I will promote physical activities of all sorts as enjoyable ways to keep your body moving, so that throughout life, fitness will be a byproduct of activities you like to do. After a general guide to the basic physiology and anatomy of exercise, we will discuss activities that make us stronger, healthier, and better able to enjoy all other aspects of life. We will discuss the multitude of exercise options available to us all, including some that you may have never considered—though perhaps you should!

The mental health and mindfulness lectures will encourage you to use your mental capacity to its fullest at every age, from youth through advanced years. These lectures will explain clearly the benefits of mindfulness, meditation, and relaxation as ways to reduce stress, improve emotional well-being, and bring balance and calm to every area of life. After a section addressing health issues specific to men, women, and children, the lectures on healthy choices will cover topics that affect all of us and our loved ones every day, such as sleep, hydration, alcohol and tobacco use, social connections, laughter, and the importance of becoming an educated patient.

The major themes of this course will serve you no matter how the science changes, and you will hear me repeat them time and again:

1. *Small changes can make a big difference.* A one-degree course change for a big ship eventually makes a significant change in that ship's trajectory. In the same way, if you start with small positive changes, over time, your efforts will culminate in a substantial positive effect on your health.

2. *Moderation is key.* Just as your body is designed to achieve homeostasis, so, too, is it important for you to find balance when making choices regarding food, exercise, and other areas that affect your health and well-being. Some parameters and guidelines will tend to serve you well over time, and I will encourage you to find the ones that work for you for the long term.

3. *It's not nice to fool Mother Nature.* There are no magical places, times, pills, or potions that can keep you eternally young, but there are many things you can do to improve how you feel and how you live your life.

4. *Remember the Goldilocks rule.* At all times of your life, *you* will have the opportunity to make the best choices that bring *you* joy and good health and that *you* can maintain and sustain.

In short, I hope to help you improve your health and well-being by providing you with evidence-based information and a variety of resources for continuing education, as well as countless great choices that suit your needs, preferences, interests, and abilities. ■

A Personal Path to Lifelong Health
Lecture 1

You can be your own teacher for your entire life. You need to know how and where to get accurate information, and you need to have a good detector for when there's baloney out there.

The purpose of this course is to present various scientifically documented options on the path to optimum health. We'll explore and redefine the currently misunderstood concepts of aging, diet, mental health, lifestyle choices, and exercise, all within the context of the clashes of so-called expert opinions. The information will be presented in a way that will enable you to make personalized choices as you seek to nourish and strengthen your body in ways that are adaptable and appropriate to your changing age and stage of life. We'll focus on healthy aging that benefits from nutritious whole foods, in combination with enjoyable and sustainable physical activities. We'll also look at maintaining mental acuity

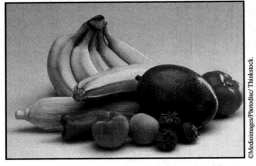

Fresh, whole foods are essential to a healthy nutrition plan.

and calmness of mind and lifestyle changes that can easily be incorporated into our daily lives. The overall objective is to supply you with a lifetime of guidance toward achieving health and well-being, no matter what your age.

You will also learn about resources for continuing your education and for using evidence-based science and medicine. You'll see the distinction between evidence-based medicine, which is hard science, and anecdotal medicine or anecdotal evidence, which is no science at all. You'll learn some of the things that can be measured and some that can't, and you'll see the importance of careful data analysis. We'll explore the concepts of

absolute risk and relative risk, along with margin of error. As much as possible, our data will come from randomized, prospective, double-blind studies published in peer-reviewed journals.

We can identify two simple rules to follow when looking for medical information or advice. First, don't accept advice from anybody just because he or she is wearing a white coat. Second, be sure that the source of your information is not receiving money by selling you the product or service in question.

We're going to find joy in good nutrition, and we're going to find a practical way of eating that will last you a lifetime.

One of the goals for this course is to find a way to live our lives with optimum health, mindfulness, joy, and freedom. For example, I don't believe there's any reason to try to maintain weight by dieting if it leaves you always feeling hungry or deprived. And there's no reason to count the minutes in your exercise program or just get it out of the way. I define diet as a way of eating, as opposed to a way to lose weight, and I focus on healthy, fresh foods as a whole style of nutrition. I also believe that physical activity should be enjoyable.

We'll return to a number of major themes throughout this course. One of these is that small changes make a huge difference. Another is the benefit of "all things in moderation." Our bodies, which are controlled by our genes, are designed to achieve a balance—homeostasis. Still another theme is the Goldilocks rule: Find the guidelines and parameters related to nutrition, exercise, mental health, and lifestyle that are a good fit for you. ∎

Important Term

absolute risk: The actual numerical chance or probability discovered during a study, presented without context, using numbers or percentages.

1. Discuss the nature-versus-nurture controversy as it might apply to aging and longevity.

2. List five common physical and/or mental changes that you believe generally occur with aging. Which do you feel are inevitable, and which can be modified?

A Personal Path to Lifelong Health
Lecture 1—Transcript

Welcome. I'm Dr. Anthony Goodman, and this is the first lecture in our series on lifelong health and well-being. For those of you who don't know me yet, let me give you just a bit of my background and a bit on what I can bring to this course. My complete curriculum vitae and training are included in the written materials accompanying the series. My background has been as a general surgeon, which means training in several rotations through virtually every surgical specialty over a period of about six years, including cardiac surgery, neurosurgery, orthopedics, urology, plastic and reconstructive surgery, trauma and burns, chest and pulmonary surgery, and head and neck surgery.

In my retirement over the past 15 years, along with the opportunity to work with The Teaching Company, I have become a professor of medicine where I teach first year medical students clinical gross anatomy, primarily in the dissection of cadavers and as well as some of the clinical correlations. I'm a physician and a surgeon who has shared the journey of thousands of patients and their families. I've listened to their stories, and now I share those with my students.

As to this course, I can say I know the body, literally inside and out. I know what fat looks like; I know what it feels like. I've held smokers' lungs in my hands. I've held a beating heart in my hands in surgery. I know the insides of joints and I know about muscles and bones. So there's literally no nook or cranny that I haven't seen with my own eyes in both cadavers and in living patients.

I know, for example, that in my yoga class when an instructor talks about "stretching the sciatic nerve," that it can't be stretched without injuring it. The sciatic nerve is about as thick as my thumb and it can only be hurt by stretching, so I ignore that and continue with my yoga. Another example: I've looked into hundreds of colons, as unattractive as that may sound, and I can tell you your colon does a better job of keeping itself clean than any program of coffee enemas or detox chemicals, and I'll talk a lot about that a bit later.

I came to this lecture series with a pretty solid understanding of the body and optimal health, and yet I did continue to learn while getting these lectures ready to deliver to you. So I know there's still a lot I don't know. I love being a lifelong learner, just like you. I have my own journey and my own issues with health and well-being. I'll share those with you, along with the mostly anonymous stories of patients and my family and our friends.

This is a never ending journey of discovery; the course is never over and I'll tell you a little bit more about that in a minute. The science is growing in leaps and bounds and always adding new information faster and faster, especially regarding the science of longevity. It's faster really than any of us can ever fully master in one sitting. I'm hoping to give you a solid foundation on which you can rely, even as the science evolves. Then you can modify your outlook as the knowledge changes.

One reason I have included a long and diverse bibliography as well as some websites is so that you can keep up as we go along and as you move on in your journey. I've always felt also that college was a place where you went to learn how to learn. The material that you got there in the first go-around is only to prepare you to go out into the world and learn some more.

The perspective of this course will be to learn about various scientifically documented options on our path to optimal health. We'll explore and redefine the currently misunderstood concepts of aging, diet, of mental health, and lifestyle choices, and exercise, all within the context of the clashes of so-called "expert" opinions, which are going to vary widely.

I'm going to present these in a way that you will be able to make personalized choices that enable you to nourish and strengthen your bodies in ways that are adaptable as well as being appropriate to your changing age and stage of life. We'll be keeping our focus on healthy aging that benefits from nutritious whole foods in combination with enjoyable, pleasurable, and at the very least acceptable, sustainable physical activities. We'll be maintaining healthy mental acuity and calmness of mind, and lifestyle changes that can easily be incorporated into our daily lives.

We'll explore a wide array of options from the current rigid exercise programs and diet and exercise. Since physical health of the body and mental health of the mind are very closely woven together, we'll also explore various ways of how to be mindful and conscious of our choices in all the areas that we're going to discuss. In the end I hope we'll be stronger, healthier, and more engaged with our lives. The point is the journey, not the destination.

I was once sitting and waiting for an aikido class to begin with my wife—this is a martial art that we'll talk about when we get to exercise—and a young man walked in, about in his 20s, in his brand new outfit getting ready for the course. After he introduced himself, he turned to everybody and said, "Well, how long is the course?" There was this dead silence, everybody looked at each other, and the senior student took him aside and explained the course is never over. This is a journey. You continue on the journey as long as it serves you.

Our objectives are going to be to supply you with a lifetime of practice toward achieving health and well-being no matter what your age. I want to give you the resources for continuing education and using evidence-based science and evidence-based medicine. The knowledge that's changing so quickly in today's world of information and the information highway makes it impossible to stay informed without being constantly vigilant and alert.

Not so long ago I was teaching a course to my medical students on cancer and I walked in on Monday and we talked about tumor suppressor genes in breast cancer. These are genes that we all have that help prevent us from getting cancer. I walked in on Wednesday and had to tell them to tear up everything in their notes because everything was wrong on Monday. It had all changed. Thursday morning I sat down at my desk, I pulled up the *New England Journal of Medicine* and they had changed things again. So I had to go in on Friday and say, you know what we've got some changes to make. This was a good lesson for them because they learned that they're going to have to be learning forever.

When I started getting that course ready, my college roommate said to me you need to change your material at least 20% every year or it's going to get stale. I had to laugh because in cancer 30% changes right out from under me just by itself.

There's a gentleman named Dr. David Sackett, who you may have heard of, he was the pioneer of evidence based medicine and he has told his medical students, "half of what you'll learn in medical school is going to be shown to be either dead wrong or out of date within 5 years of graduation. The trouble is that nobody can tell you which half."

As we go along I'm going to try to make clear the distinction between evidence-based medicine, which is hard science, and anecdotal medicine or anecdotal evidence, which is no science at all. I'm also going to try to let you know when information comes from my own experience and opinions that may not be backed up with any science at all, but just 30 years of being in the business of medicine and which allows me to draw some reasonable conclusions about things. I'll share those with you, but I'll also let you know that they are not science; they're just opinions.

I'm also going to tell you a little bit about some of the things we can measure and what we can't. For example, you're going to be presented with information about risk. We get this information all the time and it can be very biased. For example, you need to understand the difference between relative risk and absolute Risk. In 1995, there was a British study on birth control pills that put out the word to the public that the third generation of oral contraceptives had been seen to increase the relative risk of life-threatening blood clots.

Now what the public was told and what doctors were told was this doubled the relative risk. This was 100% increase in a very serious complication. In turn, thousands of women stopped taking the pills, on their own or on advice from doctors, and the abortions increased by about 13,000 the next year in England and Wales. But what was the absolute risk? What was the real risk change? Deaths from this actually went from 1 in 7,000 to 2 in 7,000. That's a very minor *absolute* change. The *absolute* risk really had hardly changed at all. The risk from the 13,000 extra abortions, though, was definitely worse than the risk from the blood clots and the possible death rate. We all need to be very, very good at analyzing data and listening to what's being told to us.

Another area that we almost never hear about in these studies is what's called the "margin of error." Very, very rarely is that put out to us, and sometimes not even in the scientific literature. For example, if you're 5'10" but you take a tape measure and measure your height, you may find it says 5'10" on the tape measure, but there is a built-in inaccuracy of that measuring tool. You may actually be 5'10" plus or minus something. That could be a half an inch. Or if you want to know how far it is from New York City to Los Angeles, you could measure this with let's say a laser out in space and you might get 3,000 miles plus or minus 15 feet. But if I walked from New York to LA and measured my steps, I might come out with 3,000 miles plus or minus 100 miles. That's the margin of error.

In this course we're not going to quibble over a few fractions of a percentage point here and there when we're analyzing data. For most of us it's not going to be pertinent. We're not going to care whether the results were 50% or 53%. I want to look at data that gives us the big picture, something we can get and draw conclusions from and then make big changes in our lives.

I've included peer-reviewed journals, which have good reputation and specialize in randomized prospective double-blind studies. What does this mean? Randomization means that the person, the author of the study, does not pick the subjects because he might inject bias in the selection of who's going to do what. These are randomized, they're literally drawn out of a hat. They are prospective because we're looking ahead at the results as opposed to a retrospective study which looks backwards in time. There are plenty of good retrospective studies, but prospective ones are better if we can get them, and we need to know that as we're drawing conclusions.

The double-blind aspect means that let's say we're comparing two kinds of treatment and we want to know whether a certain pill will improve patient outcome. The double-blind comes in first in that the author who's going to assign the patient a pill, whether it's going to be the real pill or a placebo, the sugar pill, is not going to know which the patient is getting. The patient also is not going to know which pill they're taking.

Also, when we get to the end of the study, the person who analyzes the data to see whether the pill worked or not is not going to know which pill the patient got. This takes away all bias from the studies. It would be hard for people to cheat on these and we like to know that nobody has cheated in these studies.

You can be your own teacher for your entire life. You need to know how and where to get accurate information and you need to have a good detector for when there's baloney out there. The Internet is very fast, very accessible, and it is full of false information. A few years ago there was a piece that came out on the Internet that there was a strong relationship with using underarm deodorant and the development of breast cancer. This was based on zero science. It was totally untrue, but it went around the world in many, many languages and pretty soon there was a lot of panic about the whole use of underarm deodorant. It was a bad, bad article to be there. It had no backup, yet people read this and became frightened.

I'm going to try to help you distinguish between good Internet sites and bad Internet sites, and I'll direct you to some of the better ones with the warning that they can change over time. Again, you need to be alert. In the end, if sometimes something works for you, then you may want to just ignore conventional wisdom, and stick to what works. You may be on to something.

We also want to know every now and then how reliable is the data kind of in a big picture too. There was a very recent study in England that was trying to track how far children walked in relation to the number of calories they consumed. To make it more accurate they took pedometers and gave the children the pedometers to measure really exactly how far they walked so it wasn't a guess. At the end of the study they decided that some of these little kids, and they were about nine to 11 years old, had tied the pedometers to their dogs' collars to increase the amount of walking that was measured.

Unless somebody had squealed at the end of this, nobody would have ever known and they would have used that data. But fortunately they found out it wasn't true and they weren't able to release that information.

We have some rules I'd like you to think about when you're taking advice. First of all, don't accept advice from anybody just because they're wearing a white coat, and that includes me.

In 1963, an Assistant Professor of Psychology at Yale named Stanley Milgram did a fascinating experiment. This was just at about the time that they were having the Adolf Eichmann trials about war crimes from World War II, and it showed what people later called "the white coat effect."

The subjects were told that this was an experiment in learning to see if people could learn better if they were given painful electric shocks every time they got a wrong answer and then they got no punishment if they got the right answer. But the subjects didn't know that behind the curtain were actors and they really weren't being shocked, but the subjects thought they were shocking them.

The only authority for this was a man in a white coat and a clipboard. He did not introduce himself as doctor. He put no pressure on the participants, but they assumed he had authority and they followed his orders, even when the actors behind the curtain started screaming and complaining and even one saying that they thought they were having a heart attack. The subjects of the experiment were often reluctant to give the shock but, alarmingly, most of them just went ahead and shocked the patient on the authority of this person in a white coat.

People thought that things might change that were more sophisticated. The experiment has been repeated recently with some modifications, and nothing changed. So be careful, very careful whose information you swallow. Demand and expect to see those prospective, randomized, double-blind controlled studies in peer reviewed journals. By "peer review" I mean that there is a jury of experts who read the articles and make sure that they are fulfilling all the criteria of a good study.

The last study I ever published before I retired was submitted to the *Archives of Surgery* and I must have had a hundred letters from the jury to question things in my study. I was tearing out my hair. I was frustrated at it. I was angry because they were questioning my study, and yet in the end when it finally got published, I was really happy that I had to go through that process because it made my study better. Remember even these studies can have limitations, as we just saw in dietary experiments, so be skeptical. Don't ever lose your skepticism. Demand real proof and look for the credentials of the teacher or the author of the study.

Rule number two, very important, be sure that the source of your information is not receiving money by selling you the product or the service in question. I think you should be very, very leery of anybody who wants to sell you products making health claims and has a financial connection to someone else or the company who wants to sell you that product. There are a lot of so-called "experts" out there who are selling things like vitamins and supplements or machinery and they're making money because they are touting this either medicine or procedure.

It doesn't mean that the information is false; it just means that again your baloney detector should go up and be very, very skeptical. You may just want to find a separate independent source of the information before you act on it. Use the standards of a good investigative journalist. Get independent verification from another source any time money is involved.

The course goals here are going to be to find a way to live our lives with the most health, mindfulness, longevity, joy, and freedom to make educated choices. For example, I don't believe that there's any need or reason for you to try to maintain weight by dieting and then always feeling hungry or deprived. There's no reason to be counting the minutes in your exercise program or just getting it out of the way for the day. Because exercise, movement, recreation, and food and nutrition should be chosen with a joy level that is high for you with enthusiasm. Again, at the very least, it should give you some satisfaction and at the bottom level acceptance.

What has not worked for a lot of people, but admittedly works for a few—but just not all of us—is structured, rigid weight-loss programs, tightly-controlled exercise routines. They just tend to wear in time and not allow us to continue for the long run. Mind games and tricks to improve mental acuity usually don't do that. You shouldn't be doing them unless you enjoy them. Drugs and pills as substitutes for real food are also a problem for me.

My approach is going to be diet as defined as a way of eating, as opposed to a way to lose weight, and will focus on healthy, fresh foods as a whole style of nutrition. Physical activity should be enjoyable. It should be recreation; it should be fun. The byproduct should be that you get exercise. Well thought out activities also make us stronger, healthier, and able to enjoy all the aspects of living in later life. But you need to be able to enjoy them to continue to do them; and mindfulness in this journey, every area of life, including eating and physical movement. Mental health and mindfulness lectures will encourage using your mental capacity to its fullest at every age from when you're young all the way to your advanced years. There are not going to be any rigid set of rules to whip you towards specific desired and designated goals.

The reason is if you aim and focus on losing 35 pounds, for example, you'll probably just have your mind always on the 34 pounds you still have to lose. But, if your focus is on the quality, the tastiness of the food, and the pleasure of the activities that keep you moving, keep you fit, then the weight loss will be a byproduct that just happens. If we stay focused on what is not happening it's much harder to make the change. We want to keep our focus on what we want, not on what we don't want.

People kid me in my family about my own food pyramid, which includes dark chocolate and in the morning heavy whipping cream and real sugar in my coffee, a bagel with cream cheese and Nova Scotia lox, and the *New York Times*, and it makes me happy. It's a great way for me to start off the day. There's no deprivation. There's attention paid to the rewards of wonderful tastes. I don't make this my whole diet, but I'm not going to deprive myself by putting no-fat milk in my coffee because I don't like that.

I used to go out for a lunch with my brother every now and then and I think I drove him crazy because I'd take my hot pastrami sandwich, which I loved and eat very rarely, and I would take that big glob of almost a pound of meat and take most of it out because I didn't want all that nice saturated fat that probably bypasses my stomach and goes straight to my heart. What I wanted was the taste of the pastrami, so I would just have enough to give me that taste and give me the pleasure. It was the journey. It's what made me happy and I could do that and not feel any deprivation by putting aside the other three-quarters of a pound.

Let's look at what we can all do to achieve and maintain optimal health and well-being. First, choose your parents wisely. Conventional wisdom shows that about a third of our longevity, somewhere around 35-40%, might be determined by our genes. That means that 65 or 60%, two-thirds, is within our control and you get to choose how you're going to live. It depends on where you focus. Is it going to be the genes or the environment?

I'm going to pick environment every time because I can't do anything about my genes. Also don't forget, if we're talking about numbers, this is a guess on the part of the scientists. They don't really have any way to measure this. They could vary widely. All they are really saying is that it's not 95% genes and 5%. It's not extreme; it's somewhere in the middle.

The major themes of this course, and you'll probably get tired of hearing me repeat them, are very important. First of all, very small changes make a huge difference. If you take a big supertanker at sea that's heading on a course and that captain makes a one degree change, in the first hours not much is going to happen, he's only going to be a little bit off course; but as hours go by and then days and maybe weeks, that ship is going to be way in another place than it would've been.

I want us to make small changes, not huge 180s in what we do on diet or exercise. We want to get to a new place; we should do it slowly, and don't forget that one degree course change might be in the wrong direction. You can be doing something unhealthy as well, so we have to be careful of these little changes and where are they going to take us.

The next rule is moderation, moderation, moderation. We are designed to come back to the middle. It's called "homeostasis," staying the same. Our bodies, which are controlled by our genes, don't want us to wander to extremes. If we do, we're usually fighting with our natural makeup and we're not going to get a measure of success.

One of the most important rules is the Goldilocks rule. I think most of you remember Goldilocks' story. She had to get the right chair and the right porridge and the right bed. One of them was a good fit for her and the others were not. Everybody is different. We are different at different times of the day, at different times of our life, all through the course of our lives. We can't make rules that satisfy or even apply to everyone, and even for ourselves things change.

The bed that is too soft for you might be just right for me. We often don't know which bed that's going to be until we try it. This is going to apply to nutrition, exercise, mental health, lifestyle, and there are some parameters and guidelines which we can follow and will serve us, and I'll try to find those guidelines to see which works for you. But in the end we need to make up our own minds.

We're going to explore in depth several areas. We're going to talk about aging, general concepts and misconceptions about aging, some of the physiologic factors, psychologic factors, and even cultural components.

Then we'll move on to nutrition, talk about a lot of facts and myths, a lot of science versus anecdotes. We'll talk about whole foods and not just a diet. We're going to find joy in good nutrition and we're going to find a practical way of eating that will last you a lifetime.

In exercise I want to focus on moving our bodies. I don't want to be thinking about the work part of a workout. We'll have a guide to the basic physiology; the anatomy of exercise. We'll talk about what works and what doesn't, and I'll try to guide you through programs that might work for you. We'll look and see if we can find sports for everyone so that getting fit is something we can do by enjoying the process by looking forward to what we're going to do that day to get some movement.

In lifestyles I want to look at a guide to preserving mental acuity and agility all the way to late in life. I want to talk about meditation and mindfulness, of finding stillness, of balance and of calm, of getting rid of all that noise that can sometimes clutter our brain and create stress. We'll talk about emotional well-being and we'll talk about you and your body and your environment to help make healthy choices.

We're also going to have some special sections. We're going to talk about men's health separately and women's health separately and children's health separately because they each have specific issues and problems that probably need to be addressed, each to its own.

We want to have realistic expectations for healthy and productive longevity. You may remember the elementary school or high school Latin phrase, *mens sana in corpore sano*, the desire for a sound mind and a sound body.

In the next lecture we'll begin the section on the aging process and we'll start with the cellular biology of aging.

The Cellular Biology of Aging
Lecture 2

How we age is going to vary from person to person, but change is inevitable. We can't stop that. It's how we become mindful of the changes that is often one of the biggest challenges in our lives.

The common changes associated with aging are similar in all of us. In general, we have an increasing proportion of body fat versus bone and muscle. This can affect health in many ways. For instance, older people sometimes lose balance and equilibrium, strength, and mobility, which can begin a vicious cycle. Metabolic rate begins to creep down and weight begins to creep up, initiating other changes, such as heart disease, diabetes, and many kinds of cancer. However, these don't have to be invariable accompaniments to aging. The good news for all of us is that aging in our time has markedly improved from the era of our grandparents and great-grandparents.

Probably about a third of the aging process is determined by our genes (nature) and almost twice as much is determined by our environment (nurture), which we can control to a great extent. With our fast-paced lifestyles, we have access to shortcuts, such as fast foods, that support our faster pace but are detrimental to our health. We get inadequate sleep, and we consume drugs that artificially upregulate our already fast pace. Yet in spite of all this, many of us are living longer and healthier lives because, with increased awareness, we can choose to create improved health. We can, in fact, bypass illnesses and frailties that many in the medical community have come to accept as part of "normal aging," such as diabetes, cardiovascular disease, and cancer. Many of these diseases can be prevented, slowed down, or even reversed. What is required of us is that we listen to our bodies and respond with new choices.

To understand how we age well, we need to understand the biologic process of aging. Cellular aging starts at birth. Shortly after birth, the body begins to lose some resiliency. Cells take on specific functions. They achieve specialization, and as they do so, they begin to use up their allotted number of replications. This is important because we need to replace dying or injured cells, and when we no longer have enough replacement cells, we've got a problem. Human cells have about 30 to 50 divisions before they lose their ability to reproduce. This number of divisions is called the Hayflick limit. Our individual cells replicate based on need. Red blood cells, for example, turn over completely in 120 days, while bone cells take years. Adult stem cells can replace many of these lost cell lines, but these are specific to each kind of tissue.

Once we decide not to fight aging and the aging process, we accept the fact that we will age. Then we can begin to take control of how we age.

The most important limit on our cellularity probably comes from telomeres. The telomeres are the end bodies of our chromosomes. At every replication, a little bit of the telomere is lost; eventually, all the telomere is lost and replication is impossible because the integrity of the chromosome is gone. There is an enzyme called telomerase that repairs those ends, but normal cells don't have it. Some people have suggested introducing telomerase into normal cells as a way to increase longevity, but such tinkering might encourage the production of cancer cells. We need to find other roads to life extension. ∎

Questions to Consider

1. What is the Hayflick limit, and how can it affect longevity?

2. Discuss the role of telomeres in the aging process.

Lecture 2: The Cellular Biology of Aging

The Cellular Biology of Aging
Lecture 2—Transcript

Welcome back. I'd like to begin this lecture with another rule. I don't know how many of you will remember back to the '70s, but there was a very popular ad on television that showed an idyllic scene in the forest, Mother Nature was dressed in long white robes and a garland in her hair and all the animals were gathered around. She was eating what she thought was butter but it was margarine, and she kept insisting that this was butter and they kept saying, "No, Mother Nature, it's margarine," and she kept saying, "No, it's very good. It has to be butter." And finally she learned that it was margarine, and thunder and lightning appeared and she said, "It's not nice to fool Mother Nature!"

That's my rule, it's not nice to fool Mother Nature! You won't get away with it. Our bodies have been designed to evolve and to age and it's part of the natural scheme of life. We can't change that. How we age can be changed.

For now, let's begin by exploring the physiology of how our bodies age as we move through time. The common changes associated with aging are very important because they're very similar in all of us. Not everybody is going to have these, not everybody is going to age that way at the same time, but all of us are going to eventually show some of these changes. There are alterations, for example, in body composition. We have a markedly increasing proportion of body fat, and slowly our bone and muscle begin to lose their proportion, so things change. We may or may not weigh the same, but the proportions are going to be different.

This can affect health in many, many ways. Lots of older people find that they're falling down. They lose balance and equilibrium, strength, and they get fractures. They start to lose mobility. They start then on a vicious cycle. They get poor posture, for example, that hinders their breathing. Their metabolic rate, which means basically how high their thermostat is set for energy production, begins to creep down and weight begins to creep up. This can initiate other changes like heart and blood vessel disease, diabetes, and many kinds of cancer.

The important message here is that these don't have to be an invariable accompaniment of aging. They don't have to be that way.

While we're going to focus on methods to achieve optimal health, we also have to find a level of understanding that our bodies will, no matter what, age. How we age is going to vary from person to person, but change is inevitable. We can't stop that. It's how we become mindful of the changes that is often one of the biggest challenges in our lives.

There've been a number of heroes and role models for me throughout my life and I'm going to share some of them with you. I don't know how many of you will remember George Kennan. He was an American presidential advisor back in the '60s. He was a diplomat, a political scientist, and an historian. He was also the author of our policy of containment of the Soviet Union during the Cold War. George Kennan died at the age of 101 in 2005 and he was physically fit, mentally sharp. I saw him at 95 on PBS being interviewed as one of the world's experts, still, on the subject of international affairs and diplomacy. He went into his old age the way most of us would like to go. He was physically and mentally decades younger than his chronologic age.

We used to have a saying—I guess we still have a saying in medicine—nobody wants to live to be 100, except the guy who's 99. I remember very clearly when I was still doing surgery, I walked into a room to see a man who was 99 years old and he was dying of an infected gall bladder. I'd seen his chart, his X-rays, walked in the room, the family was milling around the bed all wringing their hands and upset and he appeared to be in a coma. I talked to the family; I said look he's very sick, he's got an infected gall bladder, it would be very dangerous to operate, but without surgery there's absolutely no chance that he'll survive.

The family looked at me and they all said well he's 99 years old; he's had a good life, I think we should just let him die. This patient who apparently wasn't in a coma sat up in bed and said, don't let me die, you operate on me! And I did, very nervously. We operated and we took good care of this man. He was discharged from the hospital on his 100th birthday. I ran into his granddaughter who was an intensive care unit nurse at our hospital some years later. I said, how did your grandfather ever do, thinking he'd already died, and she said grandpa's still alive. He goes to church every Sunday and he's doing just great thank you.

I bring this up because all the numbers have changed. We can't measure things by the way we did years ago. You have to take every individual for what they are and how they're living.

My father, on the other hand, despite extraordinary genes, died at the age of 65 and I think it was because of lifestyle, diet, some habits he had including smoking, because all the members of his family besides him lived into their 80s and their mid-90s in very good health, mental acuity, and very active. His lifestyle went against him and his death was probably more about lifestyle than genes.

I hesitate to tell you this story, but my mother died at 95 having smoked two packs of cigarettes a day since she was 14. She never did any organized exercise except for running for busses in New York City and also leaving us exhausted in her wake while she went shopping. She must have had fabulous genes. I hope that I share those genes.

The good news for all of us is that aging in our time, in this era, is markedly improved from the era of our grandparents and our great grandparents and our ancestors way, way back not only in longevity, but in quality of life as well. The life expectancy gains that we have had over the many thousands of years that we can estimate, and clearly these are just estimates, are remarkable.

If you look back at the Bronze Age, which was about 3000 to 1000 BCE, people lived to the age, we think from archaeological findings, of about 18 years old. They probably died of trauma, of infection, of being eaten by animals.

In ancient Greece, which is now only about 1000 to 100 BCE, that life expectancy was up to 20 or 30 years old. By 1850, quite a bit later, we were up to 38 years old, 1900, 48 years old, 1950 now, we're getting closer to this time, we're up to 66 years old. In 2000, the life expectancy was recorded as an average of 74.8 years in the United States. Today we're talking about roughly 78 years. So we're pushing 80 years in life expectancy, a huge change from not very long ago.

This varies a great deal. It varies with economic status, a very important factor because economic status in this day and age allows people access to some health care that others would not get. Same with education, it goes hand in hand with economic status and allows access to medical care. Race is an issue with different diseases being more prevalent in different races, and occupation as well.

The point is that the increasing longevity is probably controlled by many, many factors of which evolution may not be one of them. The time period is just too short. A few thousand years is not enough time for random mutations to play a part in evolution, so probably this huge advance we've had since, let's say, ancient Greece is probably due to changes in medical care. This is I would think the key factor because it has defeated evolution.

For example, I never would have survived long enough to reproduce and have a family back then because I had appendicitis when I was young. I would've probably died and evolutionary pressure to get rid of our appendix has now stopped because people don't die of appendicitis very often, and therefore evolution can't play a role of natural selection.

Other factors probably include safety, 55 miles-an-hour speed limit at one time, air bags, sports helmets, which I'll talk more about later, and even OSHA standards in the workplace. We're getting to live longer because of our brain power and changes in our environment.

It's important to know that our bodies and our minds are changing too and they are aging. What's most important is that it's not good to deny or push against this process we call aging. There are many things we can do to chart a course toward healthy or unhealthy, depending on that one degree change, and we have a lot of control over that. We can adapt, we can optimize our lives as we age, and we can change things for the better.

The first principle is that aging is a normal process. The actual aging process inherently serves us individually and as a species. I'm going to explore the biology of this in just a minute, but for now the important point is aging is not the enemy that we paint it. Once we decide not to fight aging and the aging process, we accept the fact that we will age, then we can begin to take control of how we age.

Keep in mind the following: A significant part of us as we said, approximately a third of our process, is determined by our genes, which we generally refer to as "nature," and almost twice as much is determined by our environment, which is "nurture." In nurture, lifestyle environment is where we take control.

Almost all of us have probably at one time experienced the results of unhealthy excess, whether it involves alcohol, tobacco use, or drug use, periods of sleep deprivation, periods of over or under exercise, periods of intensive stress. Afterward we may end up feeling horrible, we have a bad hangover, we may have muscle aches and pains, sometimes much worse, sometimes serious illness, injury, and for some people it results in death.

We also see the results in people who have lived their whole lives in unhealthy excess—and I hope I'm just talking to people who haven't done that—and end up with awful diseases and disabilities which may last a lifetime, and may shorten life by a significant amount of time, sometimes decades. Since the development of an increasingly fast-paced lifestyle, we have to remember we now have access to shortcuts that support our faster pace in this society, but that are detrimental to our health.

We have access to fast foods. We have access to fast eating habits, to processed foods which have awful things in them, which we'll talk about. We get inadequate rest and sleep, another subject we're going to spend some time on, and drugs which artificially upregulate our already fast pace and keep us at a level that we really don't want to stay at. This has all exacted a huge price physically on us and mentally. Yet, in spite of all of this, many of us are in fact living longer, as you've seen, and healthier lives because with increased awareness of what we can do, and conscious decisions we can choose, to create improved health.

We can, in fact, bypass illnesses and frailties that many in the medical community have come to accept as just part of what they call "normal aging." I don't think there's anything normal about this. There's nothing normal about the epidemics that we have in this country right now in diabetes, in obesity, in strokes—meaning injuries to the brain, vascular injuries to the brain—in cardiovascular heart disease, disease of the blood vessels that feed your heart, and in cancer, and also in many of what we have come to call "degenerative diseases," such as arthritis. We'll spend a lot of time on that later.

These diseases are often the byproduct of lifestyle patterns more than our genes and we establish them early in our childhood. They don't have to be the norm. We don't have to live that way.

There's more good news. Many, if not most, of these diseases can be prevented, they can be slowed down, and in some cases they can actually be reversed. What is required of us is that we slow down and that we listen to our bodies, and I will talk later on how to listen to our bodies and what to listen to and what not to listen to. We have to respond with new choices. How we age is directly impacted by those choices that we make by the moment, by the day, and for that one degree course change over many years. Remember that ship, very small changes over time will take us to far and away new places, and we want them to be better places. We'll see that example over and over and over again.

For most of us, the fact that our parents may have had diabetes or heart disease or cancer may be totally irrelevant to our own future health. My family, which is a very large one, has an enormous incidence of high blood pressure, diabetes, heart disease, stroke, and cancer. I've just turned 70 and I'm very grateful to have none of those. I'm trying to live as much of that life of moderation that I can to make sure that I don't get any of those diseases.

Those diseases are not inevitable "diseases of aging" and we should not accept them. We should expect much more. The only thing that is inevitable is that someday we're all going to die. How we choose to live between now and then is our choice. What it simply requires is taking personal responsibility and no longer believing in the inevitability in decline and disease.

In the lectures ahead, I'm going to address ways in which we can make very doable, affordable adjustments in our lives and create improved health and well-being. We'll look at many examples of the men and women who live healthy, fulfilling lives well into their 90s and even their 100s, who are functioning mentally and physically as they did thirty and forty years before.

We'll focus on the positive side. We'll look for what we want, not what we don't want, and we'll talk about how we can maintain our bodies and our minds at their maximum potential.

Today what we'll talk about is everything that is within our capacity to modify as well as what is not. In order to understand how we age well, we need to understand the biological process of aging itself. We'll begin with some of the science, the real science, of aging so we can understand what's normal in the aging process, a very, very rapidly changing field.

First, when we leave our youth and move off into young adulthood, when we're no longer a child as we call it, that's when we start to look toward our peak physical potential. The potential for maximal strength and fitness is greatest in young adults. It tends to reach its peak sometime between 25 and 35 years old. As you probably know college coaches lose their athletes well before they ever hit their peak potential.

Professional athletes generally try to expand that window because that's how they make their living. Sometimes they do it with what I believe is the wrong way, with artificial drugs that have caused a lot of problems in our sports world, and we'll talk about those drugs later. Bear in mind we can be very fit and strong in the second half of our lives. Even if we took terrible care of ourselves when we were in our 20s or 30s, as many people do, we still have time.

We can decide to start paying attention in our 30s and 40s or even later and still make enormous differences. We can make great progress as late as our 90s. I'm going to tell you a little story about that when we get to exercise. I would not recommend waiting that long. I think we should do this long before we get to that point.

Cellular aging starts at birth. Let's talk about some quick definitions for those of you who are not into biology and life sciences. The cell, which I'm going to talk about a lot, is the smallest independently-functioning unit in the body. The cell has within it organelles, little organs, one of which we'll talk about is mitochondria, which are the powerhouses, the source of energy, the engines of the cell. The cell itself, though, is the smallest one that can function independently.

The next level of integration is tissues, and they are made of similar cells, like muscle or nerve or bone or epithelium, which is a covering cell. They're made of similar cells organized to perform a function. Nervous tissue sends information. Muscle tissue contracts and causes movement. Bone tissue supports us in space.

The next level up is organs, and they're made of several kinds of tissue which perform a specific function. The heart, for example, has muscle, very strong muscle. It has nerves; it has connective tissue. It has all these different elements designed and packaged to pump blood to the body, to respond to signals from outside of the heart, such as the brain or blood-borne chemicals like adrenalin, and it is the highest independent level of a very complex system that functions for usually one job.

Shortly after birth, the body begins to lose some resiliency. Cells take on specific functions. They achieve specialization, and as they do that they begin to use up their allotted number of replications—meaning divisions, unlike the stem cells, which most people have heard a lot about lately—which we originate from at conception and which are what we call "pleiomorphic." That means that those cells have the potential to become anything in the body if they get the right signal.

They can become muscle, brain, bone, skin, et cetera. After they start to go down the path of differentiation, meaning they become different, we use the word "determined." Once they've divided a few times and decide to become a muscle cell, it's a muscle cell and it's never going to become anything else. It might be heart muscle. It might be skeletal muscle. It might be smooth muscle, which I'll tell you about later, but it's going to be muscle. It's not going to be nerve. The further down the line they go, number one, the more restricted they are to what they become and how many time they divide.

This is very important because we need to replace dying or injured cells and when we no longer have enough replacement cells, we've got a problem. We start to age. Human cells have about 30 to 50 divisions before they lose their ability to reproduce. That doesn't sound like much, but when you think of 50 divisions, that's not 50 x 2, making 100 cells. It's 2 to the 50th power. So it's 2, 4, 8, 16, and 50 divisions is about several trillion cells produced in the process. That's a lot, but it's still finite. It's all we get for our whole life. This is known as "the Hayflick limit." Leonard Hayflick described this limit.

If you're interested in what other animals get, it's very interesting because it's directly related to how long they live. Mice get about 15 divisions and they live about three years. Humans—and we are the longest living mammal on the planet—we get about 50 divisions and we live 70 years. The Galapagos tortoise gets 110 cell divisions, roughly, which is double ours, and the tortoise lives twice as long as we do, about 175 years. These are very important limits.

How does the limit affect aging of our bodies? It restores our body in a way you might think of as a house. If we have a house of bricks and nails and windows and wood, if you took an individual brick out of the house, removed it, threw it away, and put in a new one, you could do that brick by brick, nail by nail, board by board, window by window, and soon you'd have a whole new house. Nobody would be able to tell the difference and nobody might notice.

We do that in our body. Our individual cells replicate based on need. Cells that turn over a lot—like the lining of our intestine, our skin, our airways, those are called "epithelial" or "epidermal" cells—they turn over very fast. Red blood cells are gone completely in 120 days. You have a totally new tank of blood in 120 days. Bone takes years. Brain cells have almost no ability to replicate. They've discovered in the last decade that they have some, but it's not very much, and I'll talk to that later. Heart muscle also not so much. When you have a heart attack, the muscle dies, it is replaced by scar tissue, not by heart muscle.

Over time we lose little by little the ability to replace our cells. In the meantime you are not the same person you were 10 years, 20 years ago. Your whole body has changed. You look the same, nobody will be able to tell the difference. Not much change is visible until we start aging, until we start losing our ability to replace cells that have either died or lost their function. We're moving toward a system that eventually is going to fall apart.

We have systems which can replace a lot of these lost cell lines, and do maintain that ability over life, and these come from what we call "adult stem cells," which are specific to each kind of tissue. They're not pluripotent. They are determined, but they can replace a lot of the tissue that we've lost, such as the intestinal stem cells which can become colon cells. Liver cells are terrific at it. I have removed 80 percent of a liver in a patient who has been in a car accident and four or six months later they've got a whole new liver. There are certain cells that can do it, but by and large not most of them.

Why this limit? Why has nature done this to us? We've evolved here because there really isn't a place, first of all, for us to not die. There wouldn't be enough room on Earth, but this has not happened because of the genes, because of evolution. The only function of a gene is to secure its own survival, to ensure that they never die. When genes change, they change to try to protect themselves.

There was nothing altruistic to make room on the planet and prevent overcrowding in the fact that we all, each and every creature, have a life limit. It probably came from the danger of creating cancerous cells by rapid unchecked turnover and mutations. Cancer cells are immortal. They can live forever. They have no Hayflick limit and they do not have to die as long as they have enough nutrition.

There are cells today from a woman named Helen Lane. They're called "HeLa cells." That wasn't her name, it was really Henrietta Lacks. She was a poor African American woman who had uterine cervical cancer. They took her cells without her permission in 1951. That was not an ethically correct thing to do. We hope that sort of thing doesn't happen anymore. Nevertheless, they took her cells and they are alive today because they've been nurtured and kept in the laboratory and they have led to a lot of cures.

Her cells have given us information which was used for polio vaccine, to test the effect of weightlessness in space, and many more. The point is that the cancer cells are immortal. They have no Hayflick limit, but our cells are not. We are really like an old car that eventually runs out of replacement parts, and that's one of the secrets to aging.

We have internal aging; we have external aging. We have signs that we can see that are visible to almost everybody. They generally start around the age of 30, maybe 40, at different degrees in most people, wrinkling of the skin with crow's feet around the eyes, gray hair, hair loss in men, changes in stamina that you can actually detect in the 20s and 30s, changes in recovery time from injuries. Most of us recognize, although we hate to admit it, that it takes longer to recover when we get hurt. We have difficulty maintaining fitness after a layoff.

We have difficulty in increasing our stamina, our muscularity, and maintaining leanness. There are many, many measurable losses including cognitive function much earlier than we would've thought. It's not so visible because it's overshadowed by experience, which can tend to mask some of the cognitive loss. It occurs early, though, and we can mitigate them.

There are internal changes which are less observable and are not as easy to see, but we are more susceptible to illness. We have a decrease in our immune responses. We lose stamina and strength, balance and coordination. We'll talk about how to move on through that as we get older.

The most important limit on our cellularity probably comes from something called "telomeres." This limits cell reproduction and I want to mention it because it's important. The telomeres mean "end bodies" of our chromosomes. They are like the ends of our shoelaces. The plastic on our shoelaces keeps the integrity of our shoelaces intact. There is no information in that DNA. It's like the leader on a tape recorder in the old days that had no sound at either end, just in the middle.

At every replication of the telomeres a little bit of it is lost and eventually after, in us, 30 to 50, all the telomere is lost and the replication is impossible because the integrity of the chromosome is gone. There is an enzyme called "telomerase," which has the function of repairing those ends. "Ase" is an enzyme. That is something that participates in a biologic process and doesn't get used up. Telomerase is present in cancer cells and in a few of our fetal or early embryologic cells and a few specialized cells, which we need throughout life like antibody-producing cells in the immune system. Normal cells don't have it, though, and when the telomeres are gone, our ability to replicate and reproduce our cells is gone.

The anti-aging community, people that are trying to make us live longer, think that we should be doing something to put telomerase back in normal cells and help us maintain the stability of the chromosome. I think this is a very bad idea. I think this is where you can't fool Mother Nature and you're going to get in trouble, because at the same time we're going to be encouraging the possibility of cancer cells. We need to find other ways. This kind of life extension is not a good road to go down and we have no proof that it even works.

When we come back we'll look at some of the changes that take place in our body and see how we can translate them as to what we see in physical aging.

The Physiology of Aging
Lecture 3

There was a man named Claude Bernard who was a 19th-century French physiologist, and he is known to this day for the saying "The constancy of the internal environment is the condition for a free and independent life." What he meant was that organisms, all organisms, really need to keep the chemistry and the biology of our cells, of our organs, absolutely constant within very, very narrow limits.

In the last lecture, we saw that the body's "house" has a relatively finite number of bricks and boards and that, as we age, we have fewer and fewer replacement parts. Those are the built-in limitations of our house. In this lecture, we'll look at external stresses that cause aging and what we can do to protect ourselves from them.

There are a number of basic ideas about what makes us lose the resiliency of youth, including simple wear and tear, somatic or genetic mutation, and autoimmune overreaction. We'll begin by talking about the implications of free radicals on aging. Two atoms normally form a molecule by linking pairs of electrons in their outer shells. If a molecule loses one member of a pair, it becomes a free radical, which will then seek to bind with an electron from a nearby molecule to regain its normal state. Th is molecule might unite with, for example, a molecule of DNA. The extra molecule might then interfere with the DNA's process of protein manufacture.

At the same time, free radicals are also part of a normal defense mechanism in the body called **apoptosis**—programmed suicide of abnormal or dangerous cells. There is an ongoing normal balance between the free radicals necessary for good health and protection and excessive free radicals causing cellular and tissue damage.

Let's turn to the effects on aging of glucose, the most common sugar in the body. Excess glucose in the body plays an important role in many diseases and in the process of aging. In a process called glycation, excess glucose molecules may be inserted into proteins, DNA, or fats; they form a bound complex in these molecules and may destroy function. For example, this irreversible cross-link can cause loss of elasticity in tissue. It also causes many of the problems that diabetics suffer from, as well as cataracts, and may contribute to Alzheimer's disease.

In general, the younger body heals faster and is far better adapted to defend against invasive chemicals. It tends to have better cellular nutrition and vascularity—blood flow to tissues and organs. Young people have more active cellular **metabolism**, energy production, and detoxification systems than older ones.

As we age, dramatic changes begin to take place deep in the layers of the dermis and express themselves on the surface of the skin. For example, we lose sebaceous glands, which can cause skin brittleness and susceptibility to infection. The production of synovial fluid, which

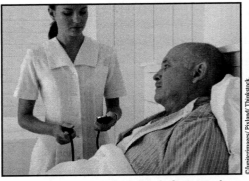

In general, a younger body heals faster and has better blood flow to tissues and organs.

lubricates joints, also decreases in older people, and the cartilage between jointed bones becomes thinner. We also lose control of the fluid, electrolyte, and acid-base balance in our bodies. This affects the heart and other organs. As a result of downregulation of the immune system, older people are more susceptible to all kinds of invasion, from infection to malignancy. Most of us, however, can take steps to slow down these changes and keep good function. ■

Important Terms

apoptosis: Programmed cell death.

metabolism: All energy processes in the body, including consumption and expenditure of energy, as well as renewal of energy.

1. How does circulating glucose relate to the aging of cells?

2. Define and discuss the possible effects of free radicals on human cells.

The Physiology of Aging
Lecture 3—Transcript

Welcome back. Today we'll continue our discussion of the aging process and see how our bodies are impacted by our external environment.

In the last lecture we saw that we have a relatively finite number of bricks and boards in our body's house, and that as we age, we have fewer and fewer replacement parts. We saw that the loss of our chromosomes' ability to reproduce was in large part a function of losing telomeres. It was kind of an inside job. So far we've dealt with the built-in limitations of our own house.

Today I want to take a look at what causes the various body parts, the cells, the tissues, the organs, to lose even some more of their function over time beyond what they would naturally lose. We'll be looking at the external stresses that cause aging and what can we do to protect ourselves from them.

There was a man named Claude Bernard who was a 19th-century French physiologist and he is known to this day for the saying, "the constancy of the internal environment is the condition for a free and independent life." What he meant was that organisms, all organisms, really need to keep the chemistry and the biology of our cells, of our organs, absolutely constant within very, very narrow limits.

If I could use a more modern analogy, the spacesuit works best. We really are in a very hostile environment. We walk around enclosed in skin and mucus membranes that protect us. The outside, though, what's out there, is our enemy. Whether it's temperature, humidity, germs, things that can invade our body, this is all stuff that our body has to deal with, and it's as if we were walking around in a very hostile environment wearing some protection.

So what is it out there that can disrupt this constancy of the internal environment? There are a few theories we should probably go through—nobody knows for sure because these have been around for a long time and there are many very hard-to-control variables—but there are a number of basic ideas about what makes us lose the resiliency of youth and move on into aging. One of the most commonly described is called just simple wear and tear, that our body cells and our tissues and organs over time just wear out. That was more what we spoke about last time, the eventual failure to replace the parts.

There's another idea called "somatic mutation." We talk about "somatic" when we're referring to body cells or body parts, and "mutation" just means change. In our fully mature developed cells, tissues, organs, we have this idea that there may be random changes in the biochemistry of the cell which leads to errors in replication, when they try to reproduce, and then inappropriate function. Our cells don't behave well because of random changes that went on probably caused by the environment.

The next related idea is called "genetic mutations." That's as opposed to somatic, we're now talking about the DNA in our genes. What we think here is that there is a compounding of errors when the DNA molecules or strands line up and try to reproduce the code that gives the information for us to make protein to function, that there may be errors in the coding and in the new product. These can accumulate leading to loss of function and even death. This is very similar to the theories that we have about what causes cancer by similar mutations, but in those cases in stem cells.

There's another theory called "waste toxicity" and I'm really not too sure about this one. It's been around for a long time. I really believe that in general our body is very capable of cleansing itself; it doesn't need a lot of help from us. This theory suggests that there is a buildup in cells of waste products that interfere with molecular function. It gets a lot of press. Most things you see in the literature, on television, and in magazines, really don't get rid of our waste in any necessary or efficient way. They don't really add anything to our body's already excellent natural means of eliminating wastes. I'm going to talk a lot about that later.

We also have something called "autoimmune over-reaction," which we know is real. Our body produces antibodies which are there to recognize what the body interprets as strangers. Anything that wasn't in our body during the time we were embryologically developing, when we were fetuses, right up to the time of birth, will be recognized as a stranger or an enemy or a danger.

Anything during the embryologic stages was fine, but anything later is not, and it's the function of the immune system to attack and destroy those. We have something called "autoimmune diseases" in which the system goes awry and the body attacks some of its own tissues for reasons that most of the time we don't understand, but we're learning about them.

This happens for example most clearly in what is known as Type I diabetes or juvenile diabetes. The body attacks the pancreas' own islet cells which produce insulin, so that one is an autoimmune disease. We'll talk a lot about Type II diabetes later on, adult onset diabetes, and we don't want to get them confused. They're different mechanisms.

There's another thing called "molecular cross-linkage," which we'll take a look at later in this lecture. I just want to mention it now as one of the many theories, but we'll move on and come back to this one in some detail. Let's hone in and narrow our focus on some other aging theories that have gotten a lot of attention in the laboratory and out in the real world.

The first one we want to talk about is the implications of free radicals on aging. If you remember atoms were at one time, when I was in school, the smallest structural particle of the universe. We now know that that's not the case. Atoms and their components normally form to make molecules retain a neutral charge. The molecules are just made up of more than one atom, whereas the atoms alone can have a neutral charge as well. Atoms are made up of protons in a nucleus, which has a positive charge, and have a mass weight. Neutrons, which also have a weight but no charge, and then very light electrons orbiting the nucleus, and they have negative charges. They normally live in different orbits and the outer orbit usually has at least paired electrons.

When these electrons somehow get disturbed and we lose one, we then have an unpaired electron in the outer shell and this is something we say is very reactive. The atom doesn't want to leave it that way. It doesn't want to be left with a charge. In these cases they're excess positive charges because they've lost a negative one. The atom, or the molecule with the charge, seeks to find and steal an electron from another nearby molecule and regain its normal neutral state. When it has a charge it's called a "free radical," and in biologic systems they can be very destructive because they search for other atoms or molecules to which they can bind or steal the electron back, and they cause damage.

The unpaired electron is the thing that makes it so potent because what can happen is that electrically charged molecule or atom might unite with, let's say, DNA in a cell's reproductive structure or in its protein-making capacity and cause damage. During protein manufacture, the instructions would be imperfect because that other molecule or atom is in the way. In replication, the DNA strands would not be able to find the proper code because the atom or molecule might be in the way. On the other hand we shouldn't look at these as totally our enemies. Free radicals are part of the body's normal defense mechanism against unwanted other molecules or cells, for example in something we call "apoptosis," a word you'll hear again.

Apoptosis, "apo" means away, "tosis" means falling, so this means falling away. It's actually programmed cell suicide. The body, when it sees abnormal cells or dangerous cells or cancer cells, has a way to signal the cell to kill itself. It's quite active, it's not just passive falling away, and a free radical is the mechanism that does that, or the free radicals could kill foreign invaders like viruses and bacteria. So we need free radicals. We need them in proper amounts. Excess ones, though, can cause damage. We don't really have a good way of measuring how many we should have quantitatively. We just know there needs to be a balance.

They can cause damage to fats, known as lipids, to proteins, to DNA and RNA. This whole big group is known as "oxidative stress." You'll hear this later on.

Where do we get all these excess free radicals? Where do we get normal free radicals? We get them, first of all, primarily as part of normal respiration within the cell. Remember I mentioned mitochondria? These are tiny organelles inside a cell, usually elliptically shaped and they are the metabolic powerhouses. This is where energy is produced, and in the process, free radicals are released. We also get them from chemicals, for example, in air pollution, toxic chemicals that may enter our body other ways like pesticides. We get them as a normal part of exercise, just the increased energy production will release more free radicals. We get them from radiation, background radiation or other forms of radiation.

When they get in excess, the body will fight them by molecules which can donate that extra electron. It can give it back to the free radical and neutralize it back to its proper state. There are antioxidants in our systems, which we can get in many ways. There are naturally-occurring endogenous enzymes, internal enzymes that effect a chemical reaction and cause neutrality in the free radicals. vitamin E is a naturally-occurring antioxidant, as is vitamin C, and beta-carotene is an antioxidant about which I'm going to talk more later. The element selenium, which we only need in very small amounts called "trace elements," is also a potent antioxidant. They can help us maintain this balance.

There is a continuing ongoing normal balance between the free radicals necessary for good health and protection and excessive free radicals causing cellular and tissue damage. In this whole balance we really need to get closer to the lower numbers to do their job than excessive ones to do damage. That's the first external environmental cause that we need to look out for in the aging process.

The second one is some of the implications of glucose on aging. We're going to talk a lot about the chemistry of sugars in future lectures, just let me remind you glucose is the most common sugar in our body. The ending "-ose", ose, means sugar, and we have lots of these and they're primarily concerned with the generation of energy in our chemical processes, especially in the mitochondria. Sucrose, which you know about, is for example the kind we put in our coffee, white sugar. It's a disaccharide, meaning two sugars joined together, in this case glucose and fructose. We'll talk a lot more about that later. Glucose is the most abundant sugar in the body, and we use it as the final common pathway for almost all our energy. Excess glucose in our body plays a very, very important role in many, many diseases and in the process of aging.

It has certain effects on cells. We've always thought glucose wasn't a very reactive molecule way back when I was learning this in medical school. It turns out it's more reactive than we thought. We've discovered a process called "glycation," which refers to "Gl," glucose, and in glycation the molecules of glucose, especially excess ones, can be inserted into proteins, into DNA, into fats, and they form a bound complex in these molecules and in amino acids of the proteins, the building blocks, so that they may not be able to be released and they destroy function. It's very similar to a process that you see when you cook. If you use sugar and vegetables and heat them up and stir them, we call this "caramelization," forming caramel.

In the body we call it caramelization too, but we're not talking about damage that you might get from eating caramelized food, because that's not the issue. We're talking about the damage the glucose does in the body that's similar to the process that you see in the cooking process. These are entirely different. The glucose will randomly attach inside and sometimes outside our cells, in our tissues and between cells as we age.

The irreversible cross-link between those molecules is what produces the problem for us. They continue to form links that cause loss of tissue function, things like elasticity. As you know, as you get older if you pinch a piece of skin, instead of it spreading out quickly again from its elastic nature, it might hang up there and slowly fold back or not go back at all for quite a while. That's loss of elastic tissue.

In diabetics, where the sugar levels tend to be higher all the time in their blood and in their body fluids, we think this is the cause of a lot of the problems that diabetics suffer. Cataracts we've known about for a very long time. It's a direct effect of the sugar products interfering with the lens of the eye and causing cloudiness. It is controlled by keeping the diabetic's blood sugar lower.

Atherosclerosis, the deposition of fat in our arteries, is another one. Chronic vascular complications of diabetes which includes small vessel disease, capillary disease, and other vascular or blood vessel diseases in the diabetic that makes them get gangrene, lose limbs, and as well as Alzheimer's disease, which has something to do, we believe, with glycosylation too.

Glucose may be a significant contributing factor to many of our diseases. Let's look at some of the other general effects of aging on body tissues and just quickly go through them one by one. The aging of tissues in general we can say in the young, for example, after injuries, all the tissues of the body heal faster, they scar less, they remodel.

For example in pediatric fractures, if you take a six year old who has a broken arm, even if it was set improperly, at an angle, in a few months to a year's time the body will straighten out that child's bone, remodel the fracture site and you could not detect on an X-ray years later that they ever had a fracture at all. In an adult if you did that, the bone would stay healed at an angle, you'd lose function, you'd see scarring and callus, totally different. There are all kinds of magic in that young part of our lives.

In fact, we now, as you probably have read, can do surgery on fetuses *in utero*. We can use small instruments and repair defects in the heart, close over a spinal cord opening in something called "spina bifida," and when that baby is born and grows up there are no scars at all. They cannot be detected.

The young body is far better adapted to challenge the invasive chemicals that get into our body and also to get rid of physical challenges as well. It has an enhanced nutritional state; they tend to have better cellular nutrition. Their tissues and organs have better blood flow early in life than later. We call that "vascularity." They have more active cellular metabolism, energy production, and detoxification systems than when we get older. As we move from youth to adulthood and then into the later years, as we age, things change and we lose a lot of this adaptability.

Let's look at some of the organ systems very quickly and see what happens to us, and then talk about what we can do minimize and avoid these changes of aging.

The skin is the most visible part. We start seeing this certainly in many people's 30s and almost always by the 40s. Dramatic changes by the late 40s, mostly in the very deep layers of the dermis, and they express themselves on the surface of the skin. Collagen, for example, is a protein and it's a connective tissue protein that gives our tissue strength. It is fiber for fiber, millimeter for millimeter, stronger than steel, but it's very flexible. This collagen starts to lose its elasticity and begins to break apart and fracture as we get older. It microscopically becomes disorganized and goes into an unstructured mass.

The elastic fibers in our body, the ones I mentioned that pull you back to your normal state after you distort your skin, begin to disintegrate. This is very, very accelerated in smokers, which is why smokers tend to have more wrinkled skin earlier. Also UV light exposure, getting too much sun on your skin, will cause this deep down destruction.

A lot of the skin changes are important. We have sebaceous glands on our skin which secrete lubrication. They get smaller in size and smaller in number. Elderly people get brittle, dry, broken skin, which is easily infected because the sebaceous glands protect us from that. Sweat production diminishes as our sweat glands lose function, and as you probably know temperature regulation in our body is primarily from evaporation from sweat even when you don't see it. Sweat occurs when we're exceeding our ability to evaporate, but normally you're actually sweating all the time, cooling your body. That's one way of controlling body temperature. We get decreased water loss from the skin, from evaporational cooling, and a much higher incidence of heat stroke in the elderly.

I went to my son's graduation a year ago from college. It was a very warm day. By nine o'clock in the morning the ambulances were arriving in a steady stream taking away the grandparents who had heat stroke even in the face of lots of free bottled water everywhere. The elderly really have to be protected from that, and from dehydration.

We get pigment changes in our skin. There are cells called "melanocytes." They produce melanin, a pigment, and the loss of that leads to the graying of the hair and irregular skin pigmentation. We get both decrease in pigmentation in some areas and what we've come to call "age spots" in others called often "café au lait" because they're usually the color of coffee with milk in it. We get more susceptible to cancer and things like pressure sores, decubitus ulcers, which means skin breakdown on the part lying down, that's what decubitus means.

The takeaway from this part is we have to protect our skin. As we go in life we want to protect our children early in life. We want to make sure they don't get too much sun, and then later on we want to keep up the sun block, of which I'll speak later, moisturizers in dry climates, lip protection, and again no smoking. Smoking is one of the most detrimental things that you can do to your skin.

The joints of our body are really important and they are made of two anatomically important structures. Basically the joints work to allow us freedom of motion. Our bones are not welded together, but can move because we have joints. There are two structures that get involved that we need to talk about. The first is called "synovial tissue." It's a thin membranous tissue that secretes fluid and just lubricates our joints like oil in a car. The second is cartilage, and at the end of our long bones, if this were to be my femur and my knee, at the end of our long bones in that joint we don't have bone-to-bone contact. Instead we have cartilage, a thin layer of much softer material that cushions the impact between what we call "articular" bones, jointed bones.

What happens with age, we get a decrease in the production of the synovial fluid, which means our lubrication, like the Tin Man in the *Wizard of Oz*, is not satisfactory. We get our bones rubbing and squeaking, and actually making noises for other reasons, and the articular cartilage becomes thinner and thinner. The cartilage gets worn out and we just can't replace it fast enough.

We also have structures called "ligaments." Ligaments are made of connective tissue, primarily of collagen, and they attach bone to bone so they prevent instability of the bones, and I'll talk more about the structures of joints later on when we get to exercise. Just know that these ligaments that provide the stability become less flexible and floppy. They can also shrink in length at times, meaning they become more susceptible to injury and they lose their strength. We need to do something about that and we can.

Mostly this phenomenon is a wear-and-tear issue with some genetic influence, you get some of it from your parents, but mostly it's just wear and tear of this body that we live in. You'll hear the term "osteoarthritis." "Itis" means inflammation, "arthro" means joint, "osteo" is bone. So osteoarthritis is inflammation in the bones of your joints. It's a disease of wear and tear, exactly what I just described, mostly older patients, mostly big joints. By age 80 almost everybody in our society has some degeneration in a major weight-bearing, over-used joint, knees, hips, elbows, shoulders. It always used to be the men more than the women, but because of increased activity in sports among women, they've caught up in that too, and that'll probably even out over time.

I'm not going to spend much time on rheumatoid arthritis except to say it's an autoimmune disease of those synovial membranes I mentioned. Our body is trying to reject those, usually occurring in much younger people. It can be as early as 20 years of age and usually in the smaller joints, the fingers and toes.

We live beyond our evolutionary limits, not because we've evolved very much over the past 200 years, but as I mentioned, because of improvements in medicine, nutrition, and so on. There has been no evolutionary compensation in our joints to match the increase in our lives, because evolution never protects us against things that occur after reproduction. Our joints are good enough to get us going, find a mate, reproduce, and after that, evolution doesn't work. We are kind of condemned to some problems in our joints which are always going to be there, and we have to protect ourselves and make sure our body is working all the time at its best. We'll talk about that later.

We also have a loss of the control of the fluid, electrolytes, and acid-based balance in our bodies, Claude Bernard again, the constancy of the internal environment. Infants also have a hard time keeping the balance, electrolytes being charged ions like sodium, chloride, potassium, you've heard these. There are lots of them dissolved in our bodies and we have trouble regulating that as we get older. By the age of 65 or 70, this impairment leads to a number of risks for us. It affects our heart and it affects other organs in our body, our nervous system, same with our acid-based balance. It results in dehydration, sometimes heart arrhythmias, and other things that we have to compensate for in the elderly.

The immune system is also a problem. Older people are more susceptible to basically all kinds of invasion, from infection to malignancy. This is from downregulation of the immune system, and their responses to vaccines are also sometimes diminished. Paradoxically, older people also may produce more autoantibodies, remember the autoimmune problems, leading to more autoimmune diseases. This is from paradoxical upregulation, inappropriately, in the immune system.

We will most likely see a gradual shift in decline in the function of most organ systems as the years progress. But for most of us we can take steps to slow these changes down, and in some cases, such as the musculoskeletal system, we can make a marked improvement or at least stability late into life.

The takeaway is that we can do a lot to slow the progression and keep good function, and that's what we'll be discussing in the upcoming lectures, the things we can do. Again the choice is ours.

The next times we'll take a look at some of the myths around the search for eternal youth.

Myths of Aging—Magical Times and Places
Lecture 4

The other philosophical view which we could and probably should take is that aging and death are, on the one hand, reverse sides of the same coin as youth and life. It's what gives life meaning and beauty and urgency and poignancy—the fact that we know we're going die.

Chronologic age is the number you arrive at by starting with the day you were born and counting forward. Biologic or physiological age is the state of wellness or illness as a total reflection of each of us as functioning organisms. Aging is a continuous process, but the rate at which we age is variable. You may be able to modify your lifestyle so that the process is exciting and productive while it continues. How quickly or slowly we age depends on how we preserve our function or how our function declines.

As a society, we have been engaged in a campaign to find a fountain of youth, something that will make us live for a very long time. This has spawned a multibillion-dollar industry that, in the end, has produced almost nothing of value. Professor Jay Olshansky of the School of Public Health at the University of Illinois described basically three legends in the quest for immortality: the antediluvian legend (meaning "before the flood"), hyperborean legends (eternal youth derived from a magical place "beyond the north wind"), and fountain-of-youth legends.

In almost every successive generation of humans, average lifespan has surpassed that of the generation before it. There is no scientific evidence to show that in some antediluvian time, longevity was much greater than what we have seen over recorded history. We also have no evidence that a magical environment exists where people live extraordinarily long lives, although there are some areas where longevity is remarkable, such as Okinawa in Japan, Abkhazia in the former Soviet Union, and Loma Linda, California. These environments have no commonalities of geography or ethnicity, but they are all clean and nontoxic, and the people there share several lifestyle factors that contribute to longevity. They all tend to have a low **body mass** index (BMI); they eat healthy diets rich in vegetables and fruits; they have low meat intake; they use very few chemicals except salt to preserve their food; they engage in consistent, lifelong, strenuous physical activity; and they have strong social ties. We can incorporate many of these factors into our own lifestyles.

The good news is that every region of the world has places that can support healthy and productive people over the age of 100 years old. These "blue zones" are getting more and more press, but we should remember that the people there have adopted lifestyle changes over generations that suit them very well. There's nothing magical in those places. We can add to our longevity by making the same adaptations to our lifestyles.

In the next lecture, we'll turn to the myths and truths about magical foods, medicines, and supplements to see what their place is in the search for longevity and healthy lives. ■

Important Term

body mass index (BMI): The standard method of determining an individual's healthy weight range by height-to-weight ratio. To calculate, multiply your weight in pounds by 703, and divide by your height in inches squared.

Questions to Consider

1. Discuss some of the commonalities in lifestyle that are found in places where people tend to have extreme longevity (the blue zones).

2. Which of those blue-zone lifestyle choices have you adopted?

Myths of Aging—Magical Times and Places
Lecture 4—Transcript

Welcome back. Today I want to continue our discussion of the aging process in general, and I want to focus specifically on aspects of the quest for eternal youth that has dominated so many societies for so long, and especially ours. Let's start in the beginning with a little definition and the difference between biologic age and chronologic age.

The difference is that chronologic age is something that you arrive at merely by starting with the day you were born and counting forward. It really doesn't have a lot of meaning. It's just a number. What we're more interested in is the biologic or the physiologic age which is the state of wellness or illness as a total reflection of each of us as functioning organisms. It's how we feel and how we are in the world. It reflects the majority of how you feel about yourself and not necessarily what you see when you look in the mirror, and this is very, very critical.

I want to tell you a story about a woman I met who was just extraordinary. I was a junior in medical school and I was on a rotation, an elective, out in the backcountry near Shiprock, New Mexico, at an Indian hospital, a Navajo Indian hospital, and I was asked to go see a 104-year-old woman who was admitted for an infection in her ankle. The infection was something she got from a splinter that had been there for a couple of weeks, and she got that splinter while she was chopping wood for her cooking fire.

She was so mentally alert that I really had to go back that night and talk to her some more with the help of a translator, because she only spoke Navajo, and she told me the story of The Long Walk a hundred years before. She was 4 years old and she walked with her grandmother and 8,200 other Navajos over 300 miles in the dead of winter guarded by the U.S. Cavalry and Kit Carson. On the way, 200 people died and she remembered every detail of this. She remembered even Yellow Hair on his big horse who was Kit Carson.

Keep in mind when we talk about the common lifestyle habits of the very long-lived people of the world, that she is one of them, and she will exemplify the kind of aging we all look forward to. It's going to strike a chord with you and we'll come back to her kind of lifestyle.

When we get talking about aging we really have to get real and think about what is aging all about and what we can expect. It's a continuous process, but the point is that the rate at which we age is very variable. It may be slowed down. You may be able to modify your lifestyle so that it is exciting and productive while it continues. The question is how quickly, or slowly we age, and much of that is going to depend upon how we preserve our function or how our function declines.

In the next two lectures I'd like to look at the reality of the pursuit of the "Myth of Eternal Youth." In this case I'm going to define "myth" the way it has been defined as stories we tell ourselves as a society. Joseph Campbell at Sarah Lawrence University was famous for his definition of the famous myths of the world, and we're going to look at these first ones as that kind of a story, not something that's untrue necessarily.

While it's worthwhile examining what's possible and what is not from the very beginning, we need to dispel some of the myths so we won't feel disappointed or cheated when they don't turn out to be true. We'll get down to the realistic goals and what we can expect, and what we cannot.

Bear in mind throughout this course that we are probably the only species of animals that outlive by many, many decades our reproductive capability. So this presents some challenges because most animals die as soon as they end their ability to create offspring. For us, we have things that I mentioned before like the failure of our joints to evolve in ways to protect us long after child-bearing age, and also for post menopausal concerns in women which we'll talk about later, hormonal changes and imbalances that drastically change their way of life. At the same time, life expectancy has improved and so has the quality of life in the recent times.

We talked about this in the earlier lecture, how for example in the Bronze Age we only lived to about 18 years and now we're pushing 80 years. That's a remarkable amount of change in a short period of time. The other philosophical view which we could and probably should take is that aging and death are on the one hand reverse sides of the same coin as youth and life. It's what gives life meaning and beauty and urgency and poignancy, the fact that we know we're going die. If we could live forever, there would probably be aspects of it that we would find intolerable. We would lose friends and family, probably lose our mental faculties while we remained alive in our body, but not in our mind.

As a society we have been engaged in this horrendous campaign to find Fountains of Youth, things that will make us live for a very long time. This has produced what is now a multi-billion dollar industry and it has in the end, after all the money spent year after year, produced almost nothing of value. I want to refer you to Professor Jay Olshansky of the School of Public Health at the University of Illinois and his book, *The Quest for Immortality: Science at the Frontiers of Aging*, which is in our bibliography.

He and several others have described different legends in the quest for immortality and they're worth examining in detail if only again to see what's true and what's not true and what we can expect. There are basically three of them. The first is called the "antediluvian legend," and "ante" meaning before, "diluvian" meaning the deluge or the flood, so it's referring to an Age of Eternal Youth or a special time before aging as we know it occurred. The second one we'll look at is called the "hyperborean legends," "hyper" meaning above or beyond, and "borean" referring to the north, meaning the north wind. Eternal youth derived from a magical place, as opposed to time that's outside the harsh realities of our world.

Then there are the Fountain of Youth legends, which are fantastic and magical substances and medicines which can preserve youth. This was exemplified by Ponce de Leon's journey to the New World in 1513 when he landed in Florida searching for, literally, the Fountain of Youth.

Let's look at each of the legends and see where the search has led us.The antediluvian legend, before the flood, this is the concept that there are times in history when people lived very long lives. Over recorded history, we have expanded our life expectancy, as you saw, from 20 to 30 years in the past up to the 80 years on the average that we're pushing right now, and about 122 years is the documented event of the longest-lived person and I'll refer to that in just a minute.

What is the maximum time that a human could possibly live? Well is it more than 122 years? Probably! How much more? I don't know, only time is going to tell that and we'll have to see, but it will not be infinite. I have really good reason to believe that it won't.

Claims have been made about exceptional longevity of people living 130 to 160 years. They have never proven out because we lack the documents in those cases like birth certificates, passports, baptismal certificates, anything to really nail down their ages. The oldest documented age that we know about was a woman name Jeanne Calment, a French woman who died in good health and fine mental acuity when she was 122.5 years old. She led a life of strenuous physical activity. She took up fencing when she was 85 years old, and I'll talk to you more about that because I have some suggestions for all of us. She was still biking at 100 and she did give up smoking for her health when she was 117.

When she was interviewed she attributed her longevity to garlic, vegetables, cigarettes, red wine, and avoiding brawls. She also attributed some of her longevity to olive oil that she added to her food and used on her skin. She drank port wine. She had about two pounds of chocolate every week! That's my kind of woman.

One of my favorite quotes that she was supposed to have said when she was 110, she said, "I only have ever had one wrinkle, and I'm sitting on it." Then a younger friend said to her as they said goodbye and parted, "Well, until next year, perhaps," and Calment replied, "I don't see why not! You don't look so bad to me." So a sense of humor was clearly there and we're going to talk about how important humor is to longevity and to well-being. So for the moment, 122.5 years is still the defined record for human age.

In almost every successive generation, up until now, we have had longevity that always surpassed the one before in terms of average life span. There has never been a period of time that we can look at that equals the life expectancy of today. That may not continue, but it so far has been the case. There is no scientific evidence yet that there was an antediluvian time long ago before the flood such as those mentioned, for example, in the bible when Methuselah was supposed to have lived for 969 years, Abraham for 175 years. Those may be true, but we have no evidence.

We do have strong scientific and archaeologic evidence suggesting that longevity of that type has never existed because we have artifacts and other fossil evidence that almost all the eras of human existence have been covered and even evidence for example that man's first neurosurgical operation took place in prehistoric times. We have found fossil evidence that men were able to put burr holes called "trephination" into the skull and into the brain to remove perhaps blood clots or evil humors, to let the evil humors out, and those wounds actually healed. Those were the first major operations that we know of that ever healed.

Maybe in the future we'll find evidence that there was such antediluvian longevity, but not yet. There has never been that time that we know of where there was exceptional longevity. I'm not going to spend any more time on that subject because I don't think we need to look to it for any information.

In the second of these legends, the hyperborean legend, we're talking about this place "Beyond the North Wind" and what we're talking about here is a place of extraordinary longevity. If you haven't read James Hilton's *Lost Horizon* from 1933, I really recommend it. It's a wonderful book. It has stood the test of time and there was a movie with Ronald Coleman and Jane Wyatt about the same thing, which also has stood the test of time. What it describes is an area or an idea that there exists a faraway place, now a place, not a time, with certain attributes, pure air, rare and exotic foods, environment that is protected from the toxins of our city. It is an environment, a place, with magic powers.

It is Shangri-La in the book and we use that term today to describe wonderful places with special attributes, generally thought to have a meditative group of people who lived long and stayed young. That was the important part of the legend. They don't age physically or mentally at all, as if by the magic of the place. The legend has it also that when they leave the environs of the place, the specific area, they wither and die almost instantly and it's all about the environment. It's all about the place.

If such a place exists, and remember there are few places on Earth left to be explored, we've seen almost everywhere, we have yet to find anything like it. There are many places that are healthier in lots of regards, then our cities that we live in. They have cleaner air, slower-paced lifestyle, but many of these places are very remote. Life is very hard, death is often just around the corner from things like simple falls, fractures, trauma, infections, venomous bites like snakes, or being eaten by a larger creature. They have local wars, which are very violent, and no medical care or long distances to medical care. In many places it's not as wonderful as it sounds.

Life expectancy in those most areas is mostly lower than in medically advanced places in the world, even if they seem to be more idyllic.

I hope you will have time to look at our bibliography, especially *The Blue Zones* book by Dan Buettner, and *The Quest for Immortality: Science at the Frontiers of Aging* by Olshansky and Carnes and also some of John Robbins' earlier books.

There are places that we can learn from where longevity is remarkable. Even though it's not Shangri-La, there's something special about these places. They are, just as a sampling, Okinawa, which is an island off the coast of Japan; Abkhazia, which is in the Caucasus region of the former Soviet Union; Vilcabamba in Ecuador, the Hunza Valley in Pakistán, the Arzana village of Sardinia, and even in the United States in Loma Linda, California, a community of Seventh Day Adventists, and Hojancha village in Costa Rica, and several others.

What's interesting is that we want to look at what these places have in common because we can learn something from them. It's not geography. They are very, very varied. They are mountains, they are valleys, they are seaside, as well as inland. They have high and low altitudes, and they also are on islands and continents. There are small cities and there are very rural. The place itself is not the issue. It's probably something about lifestyle.

There are no commonalities of geography of the physical place. There is no common ethnicity, some, like Okinawa in Japan, have a very, very narrow range of DNA because of lots of inbreeding among the islanders with very little mixing with outsiders. While here in the U.S. we have enormous mixing, a lot of what we call "hybridization" of our DNA in our melting-pot culture, and we will find that longevity exists in all kinds of DNA mixes. It's not the genetics.

When it comes down to places and societies that do have extraordinarily useful longevity, meaning their people age well, it seems to be a matter of a combination of factors. The important piece of this is that we can learn from these factors and extrapolate them to our own society no matter where we live.

First of all they all tend to have a very low Body Mass Index. I'm going to define that for you later and get into it a lot; it just means that they're all very thin. They generally have a clean non-toxic environment. They have a healthy diet of fresh foods without preservatives, by and large, and rich in vegetables and fruits. They use very few chemicals except occasionally salt to preserve some of the foods, and their diets are very low in animal fats and fats in general. They have very low meat intake as a commonality, but they're not usually vegetarians. They do have some meat or fish and occasionally poultry.

They have consistent lifelong strenuous physical activity. This doesn't mean they exercise or go to gyms, it just means what they do in this world is very, very physical and strenuous.

They also have very strong social ties, extended type communities, and extended large families that are also very close. They have access to clean air and pure water. We're going to see this again and again as we explore the positive aspects of healthy aging and longevity and we look at lifestyles.

In my youth, I wanted to see if such a place existed, and many years ago, about 35 years ago, I was an expedition surgeon into the Eastern Tibetan Plateau to climb a mountain called Minya Konka. We were the first outsiders that those people saw in more than 50 years. We were apparently quite a sight to them, and what I found in general was there was the same mix of ages of young and old, and the diseases that we see in our world and the same amount of health.

These were wonderful, generous, and welcoming people, but there was nothing special in the way of the biology of longevity. In fact I had to treat the same number and kinds of patients. We had an enormous chest of medicines with us and we did a lot of medical treatment along the way. It was pretty much the same, and so it wasn't Shangri-La.

The conclusion of all of this is that there is no Shangri-La, no place that we have discovered yet that in its nature confers immortality in and of itself, nothing to specially access extreme old age. But, there are places where extreme longevity is more common than others and those commonalities are worth noting because we can incorporate those into our own lifestyles, and then we can live anywhere and get the best of everything. We don't have to move to Shangri-La.

First of all, again, they have clean, non-toxic environments. They're usually far from the big, crowded cities, and they're in both mountains, valleys, islands, any geography. As to lower toxicity in remote regions, they may be healthier in some places, for example there's no air pollution from cars, and yet often on the insides of their homes they tend not to have chimneys as in Tibet and Africa in many places so they get a lot of cooking smoke that they're breathing in, in their fires.

They have the same occupational hazards, for example, that we have in our chefs in cities today. For example chefs that don't smoke have the same lung cancer rate as smokers, probably because some of them inhale their cooking smoke and they get more smoke than they would if they actually smoked cigarettes. They have healthy fresh foods in these places, lots of vegetables, fruits, seaweed, and their diets are consistently low in animal fat.

They limit their meat intake even when they are herders and nomads and have lots of livestock available that they drive and raise for a living. Often their diet is high in fish if they live near lakes and rivers and near the ocean.

Alcohol is a variable. They tend to have alcohol in almost all of these parts of the world, but the amount varies and it has not been well-studied.

They all have consistent, strenuous, lifelong physical activity. They farm, they till the land, they chop wood which is what my Navajo patient did. They carry heavy loads of water long distances. They hike up and down hilly terrains. They tend their animals. They plant crops, which is very hard work, and they hunt and stalk game for hours and sometimes days. We can't all herd yaks over 14,000 foot passes for our exercise so we have to look for a compromise between modern day physical activity routines and some of the elements of exercise that these other cultures have.

Where I live, in fact, many people chop their own wood to use in modern wood-burning stoves to heat their homes. It's economical, it's eco-friendly as a renewable source of energy, and it's great, great exercise.

I saw a PBS documentary once where there was a one-legged man on a bike driving through a village in Peru and he rode this very crude bike actually with one leg. He would go 180 degrees through the pedal cycle, apparently because his other leg didn't work and go back. This man was easily into his late 80s and 90s and still got around, not for exercise, but just because that's the way he got around.

These diets and physical activity are generally there to promote a healthier, Lower Body Mass Index, and much more efficiency in the heart and in their lungs.

The strong social ties and close-knit communities and the families are now known to be essential for promoting longevity in our society. These might be even more important than physical exercise or diet, surprising as that is. Also remember that we have now documented in many, many studies in our society people who live with partners tend to live longer healthier lives. One of the reasons for this is thought to be, at least in part, that some benefit comes from being encouraged to seek medical advice earlier than those people who lived alone.

This was true of my father-in-law. About 15 years ago he woke up at about six o'clock in the morning having pain in his face and his neck and other vague places in his body. It was very worrisome and he said I'm just going to lie down until the doctor's office opens at nine and maybe it'll be gone. My mother-in-law said, "No you're not. You're going to the hospital." They had a pretty good argument about this and she won, and she started to dial 911 and then hung up and just took him to the car and drove him to the hospital herself.

He got very, very fast treatment. He was diagnosed with having a rupturing ascending aortic aneurysm. This is the large vessel that leaves the heart to go to the rest of the body above the coronary arteries that feed the heart and just below the carotid arteries that feed the brain. Closing off either of these would've been instant death. They actually bumped an elective heart case from the operating schedule and put him on the table, operated, and the surgeon later told us that the aneurysm actually ruptured in his hands as he was putting on the clamps above and below the aneurysm. They put in a graft.

My father-in-law survived very well and the surgeon later told me that in 25 years of practice he had never seen anybody survive this kind of a problem. I said, "Well, how do you account for it?" He smiled and pointed at my mother-in-law and said "angels. He had angels." This is a very extreme example. He is alive and well, 12 or 15 years later, and it is certainly directly attributable to living with someone who is looking after you. It occurs in less dramatic ways too. People tend to look after each other's well-being and health and keep us on a narrower path than when we live alone.

We're going to try all throughout this course to adapt techniques that fit our own lifestyles. There's no magic formula in this. There is no special food or medicine. There's no special place. Increased longevity is found all over the world in various terrains. We're going to find ways to incorporate that into our lifestyle so we don't all have to move. We can do it right where we are.

The good news is that every region of the world has places that can support healthy and productive people over the age of 100 years old. While they're getting more and more press as being the blue zones that we want to emulate and being very, very special, we want to remember that they are special in that they have adapted lifestyle changes over generations that suit them very, very well. It's not the place. It's not the time. There's nothing magic in those places.

We can do very, very well, and we can adapt virtually everything that they can in making our own lifestyle healthier and adding to our longevity. It may be more difficult when we have something to consider like air pollution, but we have ways to get around it. We have to look at lots of our social interactions and see what we can do to cultivate them, and I'm going to talk about them a great deal in the coming lectures.

Now that we've dispelled the myths, which turn out to be not only societal ideas and stories that we tell each other, but also myths in the sense that they're probably not true, about a special time or a very special place, we can move on into the next lecture to some of the myths and truths about magical foods and medicines and substances and supplements and see what their place is in the search for longevity and healthy lives and see what we should probably avoid.

Myths of Aging—Magical Substances
Lecture 5

There's no fountain of youth; there's no free lunch when it comes to drugs, natural or synthetic. The bottom line for me is that nothing like these will stop or reverse the aging process.

The fountain of youth is the most prevalent of all the immortality myths. Its adherents look for miracle drugs, foods, or restorative substances that will prevent aging. You may have heard, for example, about human growth hormone (HGH). HGH is secreted from the anterior pituitary lobe to stimulate cell growth and reproduction. The positive effects of naturally occurring HGH in the body include reduction of body fat, increase in muscle mass and bone density, enhancement of skin tone and texture, and increase in energy level. The normal effects of naturally secreted HGH have led to a search for other ways to improve human performance.

The industry wants you to buy this stuff and they want you to use it, and it's purely a matter of money and not health.

In a study reported by the *New England Journal of Medicine*, a very small group of men over age 60 who were treated with HGH experienced significant increases in lean body mass, meaning growth of muscles, and bone density. A later study at Stanford University concluded that HGH allowed the body to accumulate more water in the muscles but didn't promote muscle growth or strength. Researchers also found that using HGH regularly brought on negative side effects, including an increase in **type 2 diabetes**. Furthermore, virtually all cancers require large amounts of insulin-like growth hormone, which is similar to HGH; this means that using HGH could stimulate cancer growth.

Anabolic steroids are hormones whose function is to increase protein synthesis in cells, causing cellular tissue to build up. Without question, anabolic steroids make users bigger and stronger, but long-term use or excessive doses can result in serious health risks, such as an increase in low-density lipoprotein (LDL, bad cholesterol) and a decrease in high-density lipoprotein (HDL, good cholesterol). These steroids also raise blood pressure, cause liver damage, increase the risk of prostate cancer in men, and disrupt the menstrual cycle in women.

Another widely misused drug, dehydroepiandrosterone (DHEA), is also a naturally occurring hormone in the body, manufactured in the adrenal glands. It's a precursor for the sex steroids, both androgens and estrogens, so both men and women have it. DHEA has been touted as a way to stop or reverse numerous age-related diseases, but again, studies have found no benefit for elderly patients.

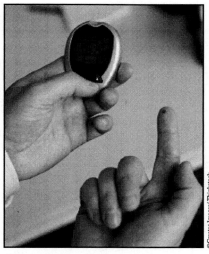

Glucose meters are used for monitoring your blood sugar levels in the privacy of your home.

©Creatas Images/ Thinkstock.

Cell therapy involves ingestion or injection of cells taken from embryonic animals, with the idea that these cells have ingredients derived from the pluripotent stem cell that could confer youth and antiaging properties. However, such cells don't migrate to targeted areas in the body and contain foreign animal proteins that can be dangerous to humans.

Finally, many herbs and medicines have been promoted for antiaging uses because they are natural, but there's nothing in the definition of "natural" that means things are safe or beneficial for human health. In fact, many natural substances that are beneficial to humans can also be toxic or fatal if taken incorrectly. Some of the biggest problems with natural remedies have to do with bioavailability—the dose and dose delivery.

Ultimately, when we get to the bottom of the list of things we might look for to help us live forever, there just isn't anything out there. We need to look to time-tested methods of ameliorating the ailments that come with advancing age without resorting to "miracle" cures. ■

type 2 diabetes: Also called adult-onset diabetes, this is the most common form of diabetes, in which the body produces insulin but does not use it effectively.

Questions to Consider

1. List five effects of naturally occurring HGH on adult humans. List three dangers associated with the use of pharmacological doses of HGH.

2. What are the pros and cons of using anabolic steroids to improve performance in sports?

Myths of Aging—Magical Substances
Lecture 5—Transcript

Welcome back. Today we're going to move on to the last of the immortality myths, the most prevalent of all the myths, the search for the Fountain of Youth. These are primarily aimed at looking for miracle drugs, for medicines, and for foods and restorative substance that will prevent aging and give us eternal life and youth. It's a multi-billion dollar industry in the U.S. and worldwide, and as I mentioned last time it all started in about 1513 with Ponce de León looking for the Fountain of Youth in Florida.

Today we're going to look at another definition of "myth," things that just aren't true. To review, there really are no true anti-aging miracles; there's no historical era or time; there's no magical place, and there are no magical substances. There's no reason to believe there will ever be, even when we can replace all the vital organs in the body because our surrounding infrastructure that helps support the body organs are going to continue to decline at some rate and maybe faster and slower for others, but they will decline as will our organs.

Vitamins and supplements are probably part of this subject, but I'm going to cover them in detail in a later section when we talk about nutrition, so I'm going to skip those for now. In that lecture we'll really examine the nutrients that are necessary for a normal, healthy life. Some of the medicines that are popular today and touted to prolong life or retard aging bear a look. We should see a number of them in ways that we haven't looked at them before because they're very widely promoted and used by many people, but a lot of them many pose great risks at the same time they fall short on their promises.

One of the ones that you've probably have heard most about is human growth hormone. I'm not going to advocate for this substance, to the contrary I'm going to point out its dangers and its failures. It's important first that we look at what it actually does in the natural state in the body, how proper medical uses can benefit people, and then we can see how the false claims can be debunked when people try to sell it to you as an anti-aging medicine. This is a very, very different topic.

Picture in your brain a gland called the "pituitary gland." It's about as big as my fingertip and it sits dead center in the brain just behind the eyes. It's the master gland and it secretes chemical messengers, which are what hormones are. Hormones go out through the body as chemicals and send signals much the way the brain sends signals electronically. So the hormones are not as fast, but they last longer. The pituitary gland, and especially the anterior lobe, which I said sits right behind the eyes, is the hormone signaler to release other hormones.

For example, there is a thyroid stimulating hormone which is put out by the pituitary. It circulates to the thyroid gland in your neck and the thyroid gland is the body's thermostat. It regulates the level of energy, and there's a negative feedback loop so that when thyroid hormone rises then the thyroid stimulating hormone falls. When the thyroid hormone falls too low, the thyroid stimulating hormone from the brain picks up again, so there are checks and balances for your safety and for homeostasis. The body rebalances itself.

Human growth hormone is also put out directly from the anterior pituitary lobe in the brain in a very, very complicated pathway, but what it does basically is it stimulates cell growth and cell reproduction. This was first used clinically when we could make synthetic or extracted human growth hormone, HGH, to give children who were very short and before their growth age was over the opportunity to attain normal height. It was very controversial in the beginning. It seems to be probably safe for this specific use, but the long term effects are still under study. We're really not sure where we're going with this, but we continue to study.

Now, the positive effects of naturally-occurring human growth hormone in the body are important because of what they represent. What I want you to understand is the physiologic effects as opposed to the pharmacologic effects. By this I mean in your body certain amounts are released at certain numbers of milligrams in the blood. In pharmacological doses that's what we give to you, and those doses are usually very different when they're given artificially. In general the physiologic part, the part that your body wants to do, will reduce body fat. That's a good thing. It will increase muscle mass and bone density, which is a good thing. It enhances skin tone and texture.

It increases total energy level and it improves the immune system. Normal human growth hormone has a lot of positive effects.

There are abnormal or disease states which relate to HGH secretion, and the main effects of the excess is that in pre-puberty, in other words before the age where the ends of your bones have closed and growth is no longer possible, but when growth now in the child is possible, if you have too much HGH you get what is called "pituitary gigantism." Patients grow very tall, sometimes over seven feet, and they have a lot of other attributes including big muscles.

It's not very common, but it may explain the whole David and Goliath story in the Bible. The *New England Journal of Medicine* one year had a lot of speculation by letters written by doctors who thought this might be the origin of that legend. Goliath was a giant. He was an enormous guy. He probably had his adenoma in his brain putting out large amounts of growth hormone and made him very big. But, one of the things that happens is that this gland in the center of your brain behind your eyes can impinge upon your optic nerves, the nerves from your eye to your brain. What this can do to someone like Goliath or anybody else who has it is now they have a reduced field of vision.

It impinges exactly where the optic nerve goes to the peripheral fields of your vision and it creates tunnel vision. This would've been a very easy thing for David. All David had to do was walk up to Goliath's side where he couldn't be seen and nail him in the temple, the thinnest part of the skull, with a rock and the battle was over. This is how pituitary gigantism looks in a normal person as opposed to someone who has been given the drug. The normal effects of the naturally-secreted HGH have led to a search for ways to improve human stature and performance because people wanted the easy way. They don't want to work for this.

The big turning point came when the *New England Journal of Medicine* published a report on a study of HGH. It was a small study. It only involved 12 men who are over the age of 60 and they were treated with human growth hormone. A very tiny limited range of subjects and very short duration. The control group was not affected at all, as we would expect, and the men treated with it experienced statistically significant increases in lean body mass, which meant growth of muscles, and increased bone density.

This was a pretty important finding because the researchers observed that the improvements were the opposite of what we would expect for someone of that age over the decades that follow age 60. It was taken out of context, though, because the people who sell human growth hormone wanted to use it to promote their product. The authors in the study did not claim that HGH had in fact reversed the normal aging process. The results were totally misinterpreted as meaning just that, this was the anti-aging miracle and that HGH was a successful anti-aging medicine.

It was so out of context that the editors of the *New England Journal of Medicine* made a note in the February edition of their journal in 2003, something they very rarely do, saying and I quote, "The article has been cited in potentially misleading e-mail advertisements. To give readers more complete information, the full text of the article ... [is] available online." So they let the readers who normally don't get the *New England Journal of Medicine* go online and see what the real results were.

On the other side of the coin, there was a clinical study of HGH at Stanford University early in 2007 at their School of Medicine. This showed that the only positive effect of HGH on healthy, elderly patients was that they added about 2 kg, which is roughly 5 pounds of muscle, and they reduced their body fat by the same amount, about 2 kg. The researchers of that study did not find any other significant factors that would signify or imply improved fitness, such as improvements in bone density, cholesterol levels, in other words fat levels in the blood, other fat measurements in the blood, or even the maximum oxygen uptake that these people could attain.

These subjects were not more fit. They also didn't find that the 2 kg, the 5 pounds of increased muscle mass, led to any improvement in muscle strength at all. That was really interesting. This led them to believe that the HGH allowed the body to accumulate more water in the muscles, but didn't promote muscle growth and therefore muscle strength. This was why they got a gain in lean body mass, but they didn't improve their performance at all.

They also had found that using HGH regularly brought about several very negative side effects. There was an increase in diabetes, Type II adult diabetes, which we'll talk about a lot, joint swelling and pain, which was very disturbing to the patients, and an incidence of something called "carpal tunnel syndrome" in which the band under the skin in the wrist, under which tendons and nerves go, got compressed and tight causing hand function symptoms, something we see in repetitive stress injury, but we don't usually see with just normal training.

What we don't see on the various anti-aging websites, the people who are promoting this stuff, was a study that was fascinating. They took 18 healthy men, ages 65 to 82, nice age spread, and they gave them all 14 weeks of progressive strength training followed by another 10 weeks of strength training adding human growth hormone, or a placebo in the controls. The results were fascinating. What they saw was that the first period of strength training definitely increased muscle strength significantly. Then when they added the growth hormone to the regimen, however, nothing improved further for any of the participants.

The benefits of going to the gym on a regular basis are safer and much less expensive than using growth hormone. Remember the growth hormone costs about $10,000 a year, and as soon as you come off it all the benefits go away so you have to keep taking it if you're going to get the benefits of this kind of drug. This is something that gets down to a matter of dollars. The industry wants you to buy this stuff and they want you to use it and it's purely a matter of money and not health.

Remember this, virtually all cancers require large amounts of something called "insulin-like growth factor," IGF-I, for growth and success, very similar to human growth hormone itself. The possible long term dangers of HGH is very disturbing to me because you may stimulate muscle growth, but you could also be stimulating and allowing cancer growth.

All this got into the media, people started talking about it, and people stopped using it as much so the industry itself that was pushing the drug tried to get around this. What they did was they advertised that their substances now, not human growth hormone, were said to "stimulate the secretion" of HGH or the insulin-like growth factor number 1. All the ones that I've been able to find are completely false. They don't have any scientific evidence that this is true and they don't have any evidence that they can accomplish this increase in HGH or other growth factors at all. More important they don't provide any scientific evidence that their product is going to benefit aging or longevity and the reason they don't have that evidence is because it doesn't exist.

We get to the subject that's very closely related and that's anabolic steroids. Anabolic steroids also related to another group that I'll use together in one group, these are anabolic-androgenic steroids or AAS. Anabolic-androgenic steroids merely means they're the steroids that simulate androgenic chemicals which means they're like testosterone, the male hormone.

The steroids basically are hormones that are associated with the production of testosterone and their function is to increase protein synthesis within cells, causing cellular tissue to build up. This is anabolism, that's why they're called "anabolic," they build up cells as opposed to catabolism, catabolic steroids, which break them down. This is mostly in muscles. They're called steroids because they have a specific spatial configuration, a geometry that makes them unique.

The steroids also have properties that are androgenic and virilizing; this means they cause male characteristics such as growth of the vocal cords, leading to a deeper voice, growth of excessive body hair. The misuse of these drugs, the major problem in the past few decades with both professional and amateur sports, everybody I think is aware of this. There was a lot of money involved and a lot of scandals and careers were ruined because of it, not to mention the health problems.

There's no argument that anabolic steroids work. They do make you stronger, they do make you bigger, they do make you a better athlete in terms of pure power. However, the long-term use or the excessive doses, the pharmacologic doses of anabolic steroids can result in very serious health risks. There are changes in the cholesterol levels, which are very detrimental. Something called "LDL," which we'll talk about a lot later; the bad cholesterol tends to go up. The HDL, which is our good cholesterol, again I'll talk about that later, tends to go down. Exercise alone will elevate and bring HDL levels back to where they should be without having to get involved with drugs that interfere with this.

These steroids also raise blood pressure, which over the long term is very dangerous and they have harmful changes in the structure of the heart's left ventricle. This is the powerhouse that feeds your heart and the rest of the body as well and especially the brain. If the left ventricle is in trouble, you're in trouble. These steroids cause liver damage; they happen to cause severe acne as well, so they have a lot of detrimental downsides to them.

In the journal *Central Nervous System Drugs* in 2005, they reviewed some of the effects of anabolic steroids on the brain and the mind. They found a very significant psychiatric symptom increase, such as aggression and serious violence, many psychoses, which means totally crazy, and even suicides. Some of the gender- and the age-specific negative effects of these steroids are very, very significant.

In men it increases baldness; it encourages breast development in the male; it increased prostate cancer risk; it increases infertility with a reduction in sperm count. It also causes different levels of impotence and also testicular shrinkage. This is bad stuff for men over the long term. In women who may be using it, also again mostly for sports, it causes marked abnormalities in menstrual cycle and eventually menstrual cycle cessation. The clitoris enlarges; their voices deepen like men's; they get a growth of facial hair, and they even get male-pattern baldness.

In adolescents, it's particularly destructive because remember those bone plates that allow growth. Human growth hormone stimulates closure of those growth plates and can stunt growth if they're taken before the usual adolescent growth spurt and then they can never reach their anticipated height, something that cannot, at least today, be reversed at all.

Also those who take illegal steroid injections, they risk the various dangers that happen when people use illicit drugs, one of contracting or transmitting hepatitis or HIV/AIDS because of dirty and reused needles. So much for the anabolic steroids. They're a really bad idea. I hope none of you will even think about using them.

There's another widely misused drug called "DHEA," dehydroepiandrosterone, forget that long word, just DHEA. This is another naturally-occurring hormone in the body. It's a precursor for the sex steroids, both androgens and estrogens, so both men and women have this. It is the reservoir from which sex steroids are produced and it's manufactured in the adrenal glands, which sit on both kidneys in your back. The DHEA levels are known to fall after age 30 as a natural occurrence of our growing older. By age 60 they're probably about half of what they were in the youth.

The people who want to sell this to you tout them as being a way to stop or reverse age-related diseases of almost all kinds, including unfortunately heart disease, diabetes, obesity, Alzheimer's, and so on.

The *New England Journal of Medicine* again reviewed this. They found no benefit in any way for elderly patients trying to reverse these or prevent these diseases by taking DHEA. They concluded that the replacement programs using DHEA were not the answer and in their words "should not be attempted." They also felt that DHEA should not be used as a food supplement, which it has been, and should instead be regarded as a drug so it can be regulated by the FDA.

They thought that the, "appropriate regulation would probably help dispel a lot of the quackery" in their words, "associated with this hormone." Regular exercise, again which I'll speak to, has been a very solidly established way to increase normal DHEA production. You don't need to buy this expensive drug and take all the risks. Once again, a trip outside or a trip to your local gym is going to do much more, be much cheaper, and be a lot, lot safer.

Moving on now I want to talk very quickly about cell therapy. For a long time clinics in Switzerland and Mexico primarily offered injections of cells taken from embryonic animals. The idea was that these cells have ingredients that derive from the pluripotent stem cell, the ones that make you young and have the ability to change, and can therefore confer youth and anti-aging properties. They took the cells mostly from fetal and embryologic sheep, from other animal embryos, and from the gonads of goats, the testicles and ovaries of goats. They obtained specific organ specimens that were thought to be your unhealthy organs that they were trying to replace or unhealthy tissues. They got the specimen from the animal for example in the ovaries if your ovaries were unhealthy.

The American Cancer Society strongly advised against taking these treatments. It doesn't work and it doesn't work for a lot of reasons. If you take the cells by mouth, which is what they originally did, they're digested by the stomach so the cells are gone. They're lost in the intestine. If you take injected cells put into your tissues they don't migrate to the target organ anyway, so they're not going to get there. The real problem is that they're loaded with foreign animal proteins that can be very, very dangerous to you.

You can get an allergy; you can get contamination with viruses and get diseases from them. There are serious immunological reactions including fatalities and it's very expensive. It's over $20,000 to $40,000 per week of treatment.

Many famous people have done this and you've probably read about them. Winston Churchill, Dwight Eisenhower, Somerset Maugham, Charlie Chaplin, Chaplin said, well, he fathered two children when he was in his 70s so he claimed this was great stuff, but actually it's not uncommon for elderly men to have viable sperm and be capable of having children. Over time, the clinics changed their prescription to freeze-dried components trying to decrease the dangers and the risks, but really it just doesn't work. Again, we know there's no such thing as anti-aging medicine

Let me talk to you a little bit about "natural," the herbs and medicines that have been promoted because they're "natural." There's nothing in the definition of "natural" that means things are safe or benefit human health. While many of the substances may be beneficial like penicillin, belladonna alkaloids which we use in anesthesia, digitalis for the heart, chemotherapy for example, from taxol which we get from trees, and antibiotics. These are natural and they are all very useful. All of them, though, could be toxic or fatal if you're taking them for the wrong reason or if the indications of them are ignored.

Penicillin for example has very little toxicity in the way of dose, but is an allergen; a very small amount could kill a person. Digitalis, coming from purple foxglove, the proper dose benefits people who have heart disease, but can be toxic for people with normal hearts, very important.

Vincent Van Gogh for example treated himself with this. He ate lots of digitalis leaves for his bad heart and one of the toxicities of digitalis is it turns your vision yellow. So Van Gogh painted pictures with beautiful, beautiful yellow hews and the doctors think it was a sign of this toxicity, digitalis overdose. Don't get caught thinking that "natural" means safe. These are fabulous drugs when they're used properly, but virtually none has been shown to extend the length of a normal life. They may save a life, like antibiotics or digitalis, so technically they could be extending a life that might have been cut short by disease, but none of them will extend an otherwise normal life.

Remember some of the biggest problems with the natural remedies have to do with the dose and dose delivery, what we call "bioavailability." Bioavailability is influenced by many, many factors. How dissolvable is the drug in your stomach, for example? Is it given on a full stomach or an empty stomach? Does it interact with other molecules such as antacids or alcohol and endogenous, meaning inside enzymes that can increase or decrease the effective dose?

There are content problems, other drugs or molecules can be found along with the primary source in a naturally-occurring molecule or plant for example like digitalis, like other drugs that we get from plant sources. Other drugs may be absent in the primary source that we need to help out such as in the carotenes, which we'll talk about later. There's the good and the bad including both contaminants as well as beneficial drugs along for the ride, so cross interactions occur with other drugs. They haven't been very well studied in natural remedies and they're very important.

Grapefruit for example contains a substance that suppresses something in our body called the "P450 cytochrome oxidase system." In a word this is the system that cleanses our cells of foreign toxic substances, which includes medication, because the body looks at drugs as foreign substances. When you take grapefruit juice and a prescription medication you may be getting the wrong dose because the grapefruit, either the juice or the actual grapefruit, can do odd things to the P450 cytochrome oxidase system, and we recommend that you actually avoid grapefruit juice – although not any of the other citrus fruits because those are okay – when you're taking any prescription medication. There's a new question as to whether pomegranate juice will do the same. I think you need to confer with your MD to make sure you're taking the right drugs.

Finally when we get to the bottom of the list of things we might look for to help us live forever, there isn't anything out there. There's no Fountain of Youth; there's no free lunch when it comes to drugs, natural or synthetic. The bottom line for me is that nothing like these will stop or reverse the aging process. We can offer time tested methods of ameliorating some ailments that come with advancing age without resorting to these.

Next time we'll take a look at the science behind some of the risks we might encounter in life and the tests and procedures that might reduce some of those risks.

Optimizing Health—Tests and Procedures
Lecture 6

In 2005, the number was 2.5 million adult deaths in the United States; that's just how many grown-ups died. An estimated 500,000 of those—20 percent—were linked to smoking. About 400,000 were linked to hypertension (high blood pressure).

In this lecture, we'll talk about which tests and routine examinations can help us stay ahead of the curve in health care. Recall our discussion about relative and absolute risk in Lecture 1. Studies have shown that a 35-year-old woman has twice the relative risk of dying in an accident as she has of dying of breast cancer in the subsequent 10 years. Both of those are rare events; that's absolute risk. At that age, a woman is not likely to die of either event, so that statistic doesn't help us. Similarly, a 55-year-old male smoker has the same chance of dying in the subsequent 10 years as a 65-year-old male nonsmoker. It's hard to make any sense of that except to know that life is a risky business.

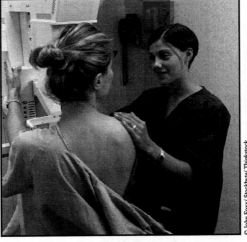

What risks can be screened for, and what other steps can we take to avoid those risks?

What are some of the big risks that can be screened for, and what steps can we take to avoid those risks? In 2009, the Harvard School of Public Health released a study showing that smoking and high blood pressure are the two leading causes of death in the United States overall. This, we can do something about. With regard to smoking and high blood pressure, most of the responsibility lies in our choices.

One of my medical school professors taught his students never to order a test unless the results would change how the patient would be treated. At the same time, we have a huge armamentarium of good tests that can help us intervene and either treat or prevent many serious illnesses. For example, in recent years, two gene mutations have been discovered that are linked to both breast and ovarian cancers, but only a small fraction of women have enough factors to justify screening for the mutations and taking action to prevent the possibility of cancer. Screening mammography, however, has been shown to have a protective effect for large numbers of women in the age group 50 to 69 years old.

For most patients, history and physical exam alone are enough to make a diagnosis. A routine serum cholesterol screening is helpful because it's easy, inexpensive, accurate, and predictive for future serious disease. Other tests that may provide an early diagnosis for diseases that can be treated include a Pap smear and a colonoscopy.

With **hypertension**, the diagnosis has become much stricter. We now believe a blood pressure of 120/80 or above is borderline hypertension. The higher number (systolic pressure) is the peak pressure that your blood vessels sustain when your heart is pumping, which gives you a higher risk for stroke because the pressure is also up in your brain. The diastolic, the lower number, is the pressure as your vessels relax.

DEXA scans, which measure the minerals in the bones, can detect early osteoporosis, which is a signal for risk of fractures. Finally, the stress test, an exercise treadmill test, is designed to pick up disease in the coronary arteries. The availability of all these tests leads us back to the need for doctors to take detailed histories and conduct physical examinations to make appropriate decisions about which tests will be beneficial. ■

Important Terms

DEXA scan: Dual-energy X-ray absorptiometry, a procedure that measures bone mineral density.

hypertension: High blood pressure.

1. Explain the difference between relative and absolute risk. Which risk statistics give you more relevant clinical information for decision making regarding patient care and why?

2. What are the benefits of the routine screenings discussed in this lecture? What are the risks, if any? Discuss the difference between screening and testing.

Optimizing Health—Tests and Procedures
Lecture 6—Transcript

Welcome back. Now that we've disposed of a lot of the myths about how you can become old and healthy through artificial means, we want to talk about what we can do to minimize risk and be proactive in prevention. Which tests and routine examinations can help us stay ahead of the curve in our health care, and in the end help us stay healthier, and which cannot? There's a lot of debate here. What I'm going to tell you is not what other people are going to tell you and there will be disagreements, but there are personal choices and issues that may be also different than societal decisions, and I need to talk about that to you.

Let's start first and talk about risks as they apply to certain categories in society, first by age group. Small children, for example, have the greatest risk from physical activity, accidents, and poisonings, both acute and chronic. For example just getting into your medicines is an acute poisoning, which means in the short term, and chronic poisoning like lead poisoning from the environment—which is what chronic means, over time.

Teenagers are quite different, they too get into accidents, but they're mostly related to bad choices, bad judgment, and reckless behavior. There's a lot that has to do with drugs, with alcohol, high-risk activities; the teenage brain really isn't fully developed. This is much worse in boys. They have the same number of neurons, but they haven't yet developed all the connections that they need and they haven't insulated their neurons completely.

We have something called "myelin" that wraps up our nerve dendrites and axons, the connections, much like black tape that you put around a copper wire to prevent short circuiting. The girls get this a little earlier in its completion. The boys do not and they have this genetic propensity anyway for high-risk behavior without any controls in place. It takes a huge toll on our children.

For men, the 30 to 50 year age group is kind of interesting because they tend to engage in activities that may be inappropriate for their ability. I'll talk a lot about this later when we get into exercise. Then when they get into the 50 to 70 year old range they move in the opposite direction, too much inactivity, too much sitting around. Women seem to be much more sensible regarding risk and appropriate behavior through all the decades of life. Their risks are more associated with things like the changes of menopause, treatment of it or not, lack of treatment, and symptoms in such areas as heart disease, again which we'll talk about a lot later, but those are the big categories.

When it comes to risk statistics, Benjamin Disraeli, the famous British Prime Minister, sometimes controversial Prime Minister, said that there were "Lies. Damned Lies. And Statistics." We've got to learn the difference. There are statistics that are useful and there are some that are just damned lies.

Remember we talked about relative risk and absolute risk in Lecture 1, we're going to talk about that again. It's going to come up over and over again. And then the other question that I used to hear all the time, I'd be sitting across my desk with a new patient or the family and somebody would ask me, "What is the mortality for my operation?" I really would always have to say without being sarcastic, for you it's either going to be 0 or it's going to be 100 percent. There's nothing in the middle. You're either going to survive, which I hope, or you're going to die. I can't give you statistics based on hundreds of thousands of people. For an individual that statistic is meaningless. I can tell you this is risky, I can tell you how many patients I've lost, but mortality has to be weighed in a whole different context, and everything has risk.

We have the other problem of the cost benefit of screening. Let's talk about screening mammography, and what I mean by screening is—and I'll mean this throughout the whole course—screening refers to any kind of a test that you do when patients who have no symptoms or any indications. You're looking at a huge number of patients hoping to find ones that you can help or cure that might have been missed until it's too late or a little bit worse anyway. We have had this come up very recently in screening mammograms.

There's no doubt as to whether screening mammography, in other words getting X-rays of the breasts in patients with no lump, no pain, no symptoms, saves lives. When it comes to an individual patient, how can I possibly tell her not to have a mammogram? It could save her life. Society tends to make this decision based on cost effectiveness. How much it's going to cost to save an individual life. I can't do that. That's not my job. My job is to treat the individual patient the best I know how for her or him.

Studies have shown that a 35-year-old woman runs twice the relative risk of dying in an accident as she has of dying of breast cancer in the subsequent ten years. Both of those are rare events, that's absolute risk. At that age, a woman is not likely to die of either event, so what does this statistic mean? It doesn't help us.

Similarly a 55-year-old man who is a smoker has the same chance of dying in the subsequent 10 years than the 65-year-old man who has never smoked. Again, what do we do with this data? How do we put it to practical use? It's really hard to make any sense of that except to know that life is a risky business.

What are some of the big risks? What can we do to avoid big things that might hurt us or kill us by screening for them and getting ahead of the curve and trying to do something about it?

The Harvard School of Public Health did a study that they released in 2009. They pointed out that smoking and high blood pressure are each responsible for the two largest numbers of deaths in the United States overall. We have effective prevention interventions for both these diseases. This is something we can do something about.

In 2005, the number was 2.5 million adult deaths in the United States, that's just how many grownups died. An estimated 500,000 of those, 20 percent, were linked to smoking. About 400,000 were linked to hypertension, high blood pressure. You add to that obesity, it linked to about another 8 percent of deaths. Physical inactivity linked to 8 percent. These are all numbers. Naturally there's an overlap in these groups; we can't separate them because you have inactive, obese, hypertensive smokers, for example, well they're all part of all those numbers we just gave you. Statistics or not, and you don't have to be a mathematician to make sense of this, this is a huge problem. This is a tremendous problem for us.

We add on to the end of this a very high dietary salt intake, especially in people with hypertension, probably another 4 percent of deaths. Alcohol caused 90,000 deaths from types of cardiovascular diseases, meaning heart disease; various medical conditions like cirrhosis of the liver which is a scarring that takes place in the alcoholic liver; traffic accidents, an enormous cause related to alcohol. And we can't forget increased breast cancer risk in women.

It's pretty clear that the majority of the responsibility really lies in us, in our individual choices. We're not pawns in a biologic game of chess. We can make our own moves and then we have to take responsibility for them.

You as the patient and your medical team, together, have to make decisions on a somewhat different scale, with different criteria than those made in huge studies that affect society more than the individual. I'm going to talk more later about the physician/patient collaboration and the medical team you want to put together.

When we look at societal choices in the allocation of health care dollars we might end up with a two-tiered system which really disturbs me, and it's going to be to the detriment of the lower income patients. For example, when the government decides, let's say, to stop paying for screening tests like mammograms in certain patients, then patients who can afford to pay for themselves are going to get one kind of care, and the patients who cannot are going to get another. That's two-tier medicine. That's something we don't want to have in this country.

What are the benefits of routine screenings? What should you consider and what should you not consider doing? Again, just keep in mind "screening" means no signs or symptoms. This is in the patient who's totally normal and we just want to find and pick them out of the group to see who we can help. Let's talk about several of the factors that come into play.

One of my favorite professors in medical school was Dr. Elliot Hochstein who was an internist, a wonderful man, and introduced us into clinical medicine and how to approach the patient with history and physical. He told us never to order a test unless it would change what you do for your patient.

For example if you have a patient who's 92 years old, he's dying of let's say terminal Non-Hodgkin's' lymphoma, a very serious cancer, you wouldn't order an HIV/AIDS test on this patient even though those two diseases are linked because it's not going to give you any information. You're not going to do anything different for this patient than you would if you didn't know whether he has AIDS, except being careful about how you handle blood. However, you should be doing that anyway for all patients today.

I had the same experience when I was in medical school. I developed measles, which I think I caught from one of the children in the pediatric ward. I got very, very sick and I ended up with hepatitis from the measles and was put in the hospital. One morning I found myself on a gurney on the way down to the surgical suite and asked the nurse where I was going and she said well for your liver biopsy.

I said, whoa, wait a minute, and I had the doctors called in and they said, yeah we want to get a liver biopsy to prove you have hepatitis. I said, "But Dr. Hochstein told us if you can't do anything about it, why do the biopsy. There's no cure for measles/hepatitis." I'd been reading my textbook, and they were very annoyed, but we went back to my room and I never got my biopsy. As you can see I did recover without it, but it made a very important point to me.

At the same time we don't want the Ghost Of Risk to freeze us into inaction. We do have a huge armamentarium of really good tests that can help us intervene and either treat or prevent a lot of serious illnesses, and we have to use them when we can and when we should. Sometimes we get information we don't know what to do with it and that's a real problem.

For example, in women's breast cancer, this is a big dilemma. Women who have a family history of breast cancer have a very relatively low risk of getting breast cancer themselves. Most women, at least 80% of them, who have that family history are not going to get breast cancer, and conversely most women who do have breast cancer, about 80%, have no family history. How do we make sense of taking a family history from a patient and what we should do for her surveillance. I'm not going to treat a breast cancer patient any differently if I suspect that she may have it because she has a family history or give her less surveillance because she didn't have a family history. It doesn't change the way we approach that patient.

In recent years we've discovered two gene mutations. There are things called "tumor suppressor genes," which help your body naturally fight off cancer and prevent you from getting it. We discovered two called BRCA1, breast cancer 1 and breast cancer 2, BRCA2 gene mutations. The normal ones help prevent it and the mutations lose that prevention. These tumor suppressor gene mutations are strongly linked to both breast and ovarian cancers, but what do we do with the information once we know about it?

We are not going to be less careful with the women who have normal BRCA1/2 genes because they can still get breast cancer, but we have the opportunity in some patients to at least discuss the preventative removal of the breast, prophylactic mastectomy, or removal of ovaries. A very small fraction probably, less than 5 percent, have enough factors to justify even the discussion of this kind of radical approach to the prevention of cancer.

If they have a family history that includes a mother, let's say, who had breast cancer at a very young age, premenopausal; who had breast cancer in both breasts, who had it for several generations, grandmother, great-grandmother. That woman then starts to move into where we may want to look more closely and where we may then want to see does she have biopsy changes that are suspicious. Does she have mutations in the BRCA1/2 genes? Most women, probably close to 95 percent, don't face this decision at all. Do we want to get this very expensive and really perplexing test as routine screening?

If we move on and we look at another link between colon cancer and breast cancer, the story is a little different. Women who would ordinarily be considered too young to start having a colonoscopy, and that's where we take a flexible instrument, insert it through the rectum, and we can now look at the entire six feet of colon. Women who might not be having that test as a screening function might reconsider it once they have breast cancer because there's a strong link between the two. So there's a good case where you might want to change your criteria for screening.

Having said that, let's go back and look at this big discussion about screening mammography for all women. We know it can find early, small, curable cancers. The important question is, does the screening with mammograms decrease the breast cancer mortality? Does that death rate change after we've discovered them earlier than we would have if we didn't do the mammography?

If we review the studies, we find that in nine randomized, controlled, prospective trials of over 650,000 women—that's a big study—for the women who are 50 years and older, every single trial has demonstrated a protective effect of screening mammography. After seven years, there was about a 34 percent decrease in breast cancer mortality, and that reduced mortality came with almost no increase in risk and at quite an acceptable economic cost.

Other data also suggest that screening mammography will decrease breast cancer mortality overall in the whole population. Women in the age 50 to 69 years old there's a strong agreement about routine screening. It starts to fall off after about 70 to 80 in terms of agreement because that's when breast cancer starts to fall off in its incidence too. The real question comes in about screening women between 40 and 49 years old, and also those over the age of 70. There is much, much less consensus on that.

Right now, screening mammography in women under 50 is controversial, no question about it. The mammography done during that time span is less likely to catch early breast cancers at a curable stage because the breast is much denser. There's more breast tissue and less fat and it makes it harder to see those cancers by X-ray. The higher breast density then gets us into some more biopsies that we might not have done because those biopsies come from equivocal findings on the X-ray so we end up with more false positives on the X-ray leading to biopsies.

The biopsy is a low risk, low morbidity risk, very few complications, but still it's a procedure nobody wants to have. Also, not as many women under the age of 50 benefit from screening because they in general are not as likely to have breast cancer. Breast cancer starts to peak much later, so because they're not as likely to have breast cancer and because of these false positives, the cost of screening mammography per year of life saved, which is what the government is going to look at, has risen to more than $100,000 per person. This is again a societal difference that we're going to have to deal with. Somebody is going to have to make the decision as to who's going to pay for this if we want to do it.

The expert groups in the meantime have recommended mammography by age, all women 50 and older, the controversy remains for the younger women. In Europe they have now started to move ahead to be more restrictive, leaning toward cost effectiveness for the lives saved, looking not at diagnosis, but overall mortality. For me, sitting at my desk across from a family and a woman who is having questions about this, I have to recommend screening. There's nothing I can tell her that would change that for the individual patient.

Let's move on now and talk about something else and that is routine screening in the asymptomatic patient. William Osler, one of the great early founders of physical diagnosis and treating patients in our country said, "Listen to the patient, and they will tell you the diagnosis." About 80 percent of our diagnosis can be made on history alone. Good solid medical detective work will pick up some more, in other words asking good questions, leading the patient to answer questions they might not have thought of. Add physical examination to that and the diagnostic rate might go up another 5 or 10 percent into the 90s. The rest of the lab work and X-rays is usually just confirmatory.

A patient walks into my office telling me that they have pain right here in their right upper quadrant under the rib. The pain goes around to the shoulder blade in the back, that they get this pain intermittently after fatty foods, that they do a lot of burping, that they are female, they are overweight, and they've had several children, and that when I push there in my physical exam they're exquisitely tender. I know with 98% certainty that this patient is going to have their gallbladder out. I will get the X-rays and I'll get confirmation, but most of the patients we know are going to have this taken care of surgically and we don't need any further tests.

That's the case for most of our diagnoses. History and physical alone is enough. When you go to routine blood testing we have some criteria that we should accept before we screen people with routine blood tests. In other words you may go to your doctor once a year and say, should I get blood tests? We want to know several things. We want to know if there are significant risks of disease if the screening tests were omitted and the disease untreated. For example high cholesterol, that's a perfect example. If you don't know you have high cholesterol it's picked up on screening, most of us don't know, then we can do something about that.

We also want to know if an abnormality is highly endemic. That means running at a high level in an otherwise apparently-healthy population. That would include for example high blood pressure in African Americans who live in America. We want to look at that population because that's important to find early. An early diagnosis could be detected before symptoms appear, that's another criteria; diabetes, high cholesterol, Pap smears, scrapings of the uterine cervix looking for cancer. This gets us early detection in treatable disease. We want to know treatment is available.

We don't want to do screening tests for something we can't cure. For example, although it's uncommon you probably have all heard about Lou Gehrig's Disease, amyotrophic lateral sclerosis, which is a neurologic disease uniformly fatal, kills everybody in a short period of time, and we have no treatment. There's no point in screening for it if there's nothing we can do about it.

We also have blood screening of which there is some debate. We have general broad guidelines including a wide range of measurements that have a very low yield. Serum cholesterol is in its own category. It's a good example of screening because it's easy; it's inexpensive; it's accurate. It's predictive for future serious disease. It has effective treatment if the tests are abnormal, like diet or putting them on statin drugs, and we have good science to show the effectiveness of treatment. The debate really revolves around who and when, not if. The other aspect of this is children, we don't know whether we should be screening children or not.

Colon cancer is another one where we really have good evidence that we should be screening. We can test for blood in the feces, very cheap and definitely increases our ability to diagnose colon cancer early.

Colonoscopy, looking into the colon with the instrument that I mentioned earlier, gives us a big jump on colon cancer because they almost all start in a little lollipop-shaped piece of the lining of the colon called a "polyp." The cancers generally start there and there's usually a polyp for a few years before there's any cancer. We can reach in and snare those out with almost no complication or morbidity rate and prevent cancers from even starting. We can find earlier ones before they have symptoms, so that once routine colonoscopy was introduced into the country, we saw a tremendous drop in the incidence of colon cancers because we're getting them out earlier. It's expensive, it's mildly invasive and undignified, but it's a terrific test.

Chest X-rays, we don't know. It's not a great yield. Remember we're not talking about a patient who is coughing or having chest pain, because that's not screening. We're talking about all of you out there who are sitting there very happy, should you be getting a once a year or once every five year chest X-ray. In reality, most lung cancers, which is what we're looking for, are incurable in the beginning. We can make a minimal difference in mortality by adding that to the routine.

The last one I'll probably talk to you about is hypertension, which we call "The Silent Killer." It is a silent killer because most people don't know they have it. There is good, easy, accurate, virtually cost-free screening for high blood pressure and there's good treatment. This is a real killer. This changes the strain on our heart, changes our vessels, changes our brains, and we can treat this relatively easily. There are guidelines and the diagnosis of hypertension has become much stricter. We now believe that if you have a blood pressure of 120/80 or above, that this is borderline hypertension. We're much more aggressive. The 120 is the number that is the peak pressure that your blood vessels sustain when your heart is pumping, and this gives you a higher risk for stroke because the pressure is also up in your brain. The diastolic, the lower number, is the pressure as your vessels relax. It has to do with elasticity and this elasticity is a signal or a sign of the state of your vessels. We'll talk more about that a little later. We're getting much, much more aggressive in treating hypertension, and we'll talk about those guidelines.

Finally, I want to talk about the DEXA scans or the DEX scan, and this has to do with the density of our bones. It stands for "Dual Energy X-ray Absorptiometry." DEXA is a better way or DEX. It measures the minerals in the bones, and we're looking for osteoporosis or low bone mass density, which is a signal for early risk of fractures, very common in women.

It's probably the most useful of the scans in clinical practice because it gives us an early start on osteoporosis and the danger of fractures. Hip fractures in elderly women are very significant, as they are in men. They have a very high mortality because of the treatment necessary, and we'll talk about how we can prevent those when we get on to exercise and nutrition and also the women's sections on women's health. There are effective treatments, there is effective prevention. It makes great sense.

And before we quit I would like to also mention the Exercise Treadmill Test, sometimes called the "Stress Test." This is a test that's designed to pick up disease in the coronary arteries in which there are no clinical findings. The patient is not having chest pain, they're not short of breath. They seem to be okay. We're looking for someone who has narrowing in the coronary arteries that are not yet apparent, but may show itself the next time by the patient being dead on the floor. We want to be able to get in there and repair that before that happens.

Remember I talked about the heart squeezing and giving you a systolic flow of blood and then a diastolic relaxation. It turns out that the heart gets its own blood supply during relaxation because when it's squeezing down and giving blood to the rest of the body it's squeezed too tight for its own blood supply. The heart is very efficient. The squeezing cycle is very short. The relaxation cycle is about three times as long, but when we increase our heart rate as we do in exercise, we can only shorten the squeezing cycle by a little bit, so who loses out? The relaxation cycle and the blood flow to the heart.

It may be reduced by half or even three-quarters the time, and in a patient who is normally asymptomatic but has significant narrowing of their coronary arteries, we might be able to show that they've got a problem and bring out the symptoms. We do this on a treadmill with a cardiologist, intravenous line running for medications, a blood pressure cuff, an EKG, and then we keep raising the treadmill, working the patient harder and harder.

Then there are a number of technical ways we can tell including radioactive die injections into the heart, echocardiograms to see how the left ventricle is pumping, but in the end we're looking for that patient who might be saved because we found a lesion that was about to close off, an artery that was about to stop flowing to the heart, before they get into real trouble. They are not foolproof; they do miss some sick people. You all remember Tim Russert who died rather suddenly a short time after he had what looked like a normal exercise stress test. We do, though, pick up some of these lesions and we save a lot of lives.

This is one I would like to see left in the armamentarium. All of these findings lead us back to the importance and the need for doctors to take detailed history and physical examinations and then follow up with tests as appropriate.

Next time we'll take a look at what we can do to prevent the illness or the disease in the first place.

Optimizing Health—Prevention
Lecture 7

Now let's talk about high blood pressure. … What we need for all of us is very, very aggressive surveillance. In other words, we need to just take people's blood pressure. It's very cheap. It's very easy. It's very accurate, and it's available. You can take your own blood pressure.

In this lecture, we'll look at some measures we can take to prevent illness before it starts. Prevention is always preferable to trying to cure an existing disease.

First, if you smoke now, you need to stop. Worldwide tobacco-related deaths exceeded 5 million per year in 2008 and are expected to reach about 8 million per year by 2030. In addition to the expected 220,000 new cases of lung cancer in 2009, smoking also causes cancers of the

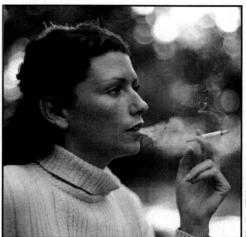

Cigarrette smoking is one of the leading preventable causes of early death.

©Stockbyte/Thinkstock.

neck, tongue, larynx, esophagus, and bladder, along with heart attacks and strokes. There is no question that avoiding any exposure to tobacco smoke—firsthand, secondhand, and now, thirdhand—is the single most effective measure worldwide in terms of reducing this morbidity and mortality. Besides the loss of life and the morbidity, smoking imposes an enormous cost on our society. It costs the United States more than $200 billion a year in lost productivity and another $95 billion in health-care expenditures. If you're a smoker, the American Cancer Society and other organizations have many resources to help you stop.

A final word about smoking in relation to hypertension: Tobacco products increase sympathetic nervous system activity, which is the part of the nervous system that releases adrenalin. The resulting fight/flight reaction increases the oxygen consumption of the heart muscle, along with the heart rate and force of contraction. Over time, this causes stiffening of the arteries, which can last for decades. Stopping smoking can lower the risk of coronary artery heart disease by 33 percent in a relatively short period of time, even if you have smoked for a long time.

Much of the research dollars that we're spending on lung cancer alone today, in my opinion, would be much better spent if we could just get people to stop smoking or never start.

High blood pressure is known as the silent killer. As mentioned earlier, acceptable blood pressure is now about 120/80. If you have hypertension, reducing your salt intake can make a significant difference; it may be the only thing necessary to get your pressure back to a more acceptable level. Exercise, weight loss, changes in nutritional choices, and reduction of alcohol intake are also well known to reduce blood pressure.

Immunizations are also important in preventing disease and maintaining optimum health. About 50,000 Americans a year, mostly adults, die from vaccine-preventable diseases. Vaccines in adults could prevent about 80 percent of all influenza deaths, about 60 percent of deaths from pneumococcal infections, and 90 percent of hepatitis deaths. The National Immunization Program, which is primarily for children, has made tremendous gains in public health. Readily available vaccines for the general adult population include those for pneumonia, influenza, and shingles.

Interestingly, good dental care can be a factor in preventing heart disease, which can be caused by infections in the mouth. Of course, brushing, flossing, and getting regular dental checkups are preventive measures you can take in this regard.

Finally, hearing loss, which can be psychologically damaging, can be prevented by avoiding chronic exposure to high levels of noise. Treatment for hearing loss includes hearing aids and surgery. Parents are especially urged to protect their children from trauma to the nerves within the ears by ensuring that MP3 players are turned down to appropriate levels. ■

1. List five reasons why quitting smoking will improve one's health.

2. What is the relationship between the frequency of cancer and aging? Name two cancers where age might be factor.

3. How have immunizations and vaccinations affected the human lifespan worldwide? Have the controversies that have arisen around these topics been resolved?

Optimizing Health—Prevention
Lecture 7—Transcript

Welcome back to our lecture series. Today we're going to take a look at some of the measures we can take to prevent illness and diseases before they even start. Prevention is always preferable as a starting place compared to trying to cure an existing disease. We also want to consider some of the resources that can keep us up to date as things change in the world of medicine because they change very, very quickly.

The first one I'm going to come back to is smoking. You just need to stop smoking if you're smoking now. There's no argument about it. It's one of the worst things that you can be doing for your health. This was established as early as 1952, almost 60 years ago, that smoking causes lung cancer as well as a myriad of other diseases, including chronic lung diseases that aren't cancer and coronary artery disease as well. No matter what the tobacco industry had been saying up to that time, it was now proven to be the case.

A couple of definitions; firsthand smoke, as you probably all know, is the smoke that you get when you're smoking a cigarettes. It goes directly into your lungs, your mouth, and your bloodstream. Secondhand smoke is the smoke that's in the air as you or the smoker exhales it and another person then breathes in after it has been diluted a little bit in the air. It's what you smell when you walk into a room as well where there's been smoking.

Thirdhand smoke is kind of a new term, a new category that's becoming very important. It includes tobacco products, gases and particles, and chemical molecules that get carried into the environment and attached to dust, to carpets, to hair, clothing, exposed surfaces, and that then remains in that environment for very long periods of time after the airborne smoke is gone. Apparently some of the residues in cigarette smoke may be worse now than ever. They've just changed the chemicals in the tobacco, but they have not made it any safer.

The undeniable part of all of this is that quitting any exposure to tobacco smoke, first and secondhand, and now thirdhand smoke is the single most effective preventive measure in the United States and worldwide in terms of reducing an enormous problem with morbidity. Which again means the nonlethal complications, things like lung cancer itself, emphysema, which is a dilatation of the breathing spaces in the lung that gives you poor exchange of your air, and peripheral vascular disease, the small vessels in your arms and your legs.

Again we'll be comparing morbidity, which I just mentioned, to the mortality, which is the death rate. The recent Center for Disease Control numbers are very, very startling. The morbidity and mortality linked to using tobacco, and we're talking about all tobacco-associated diseases, is enormous. Worldwide tobacco-related deaths exceeded 5 million per year in the last several years and it has been increasing. They expect it to reach about 8 million deaths per year by the year 2030. This is an enormous problem and it is the number one preventable cause of death in the United States today.

In this country tobacco-related deaths reached about 440,000 deaths per year, that's about 20 percent of all deaths. Fifty thousand of these deaths come from secondhand smoke, people who are not even smokers themselves. The smoker's lifespan is reduced somewhere in the neighborhood of about 14 years shorter than nonsmokers. For every death that's smoking-related, 20 more people can have one or more serious smoking-related illnesses.

The lung cancer mortality, again numbers that may be hard to listen to over and over again, but I think they're so important. In the year 2009, we expect about 220,000 new cases of lung cancer. We expect about 160,000 deaths. That doesn't mean we had 60,000 people cured because that 160,000 deaths came from cases that were diagnosed long ago and are only now coming to the end of their lives. Of these 220,000 deaths, we might expect as many as 20,000 of them to die by the time they come to the next few years, and that's just lung cancer.

We have head and neck cancers, tongue, floor of the mouth, larynx. We have esophageal cancers, which are highly incurable. We have bladder cancers that come from the tobacco products getting into the urine and lying against the bladder lining for long periods of time in the urine, plus the deaths from cardiovascular causes, meaning heart attacks and other cardiovascular diseases such as strokes. Much of the research dollars that we're spending on lung cancer alone today, in my opinion, would be much better spent if we could just get people to stop smoking or never start.

We have not made much progress. We do not think that dollar for dollar we're getting very much, as they say, bang for our buck in research. We probably should be getting people to not even begin. Stopping smoking even after decades of use can improve both your heart and your lung function. After somewhere about 20 or 25 years we believe that the cancer risk, lung cancer, returns slowly to nearly the same as in a non-smoker. It's not always the case, there are exceptions.

My big brother smoked from the time he was about 15, two packs a day for 30 years. I pleaded with him to stop. I finally got him to stop after about 30 years of smoking and 30 years later it caught up with him, and within a year he had died of lung cancer. Consequently, not everybody is going to get the benefit, but many, many will if they just stop.

Besides the tragic loss of life and the morbidity and bad things that happen to smokers, we have an enormous cost to our society. It is more than $200 billion a year in lost productivity alone, people who can no longer work for example and are out of work for various illnesses. We lose about $95 billion. In healthcare expenditures another $95 billion, and in health care costs associated with secondhand smoke, somewhere between probably $190 and $200 billion.

In the year 2005, at the other side of this coin, the tobacco industry spent almost $14 billion, which is $35 million a day, to advertise their products. In 1968, some of you will remember the Virginia Slims, the Philip Morris cigarette that came into being and their advertisement was, "You've come a long way, Baby." This was followed in the appropriate number of years that it takes to get cancer by a very sharp increase in lung cancer and death in women from lung cancer. The lung cancer deaths finally surpassed breast cancer deaths, even though there were fewer cases of lung cancer because that disease is so much more lethal. While women continue to get more breast cancer than they did lung cancer, they died much more frequently from lung cancer.

There are about $19 billion available from tobacco excise taxes and tobacco industry legal settlements that are available to the states. Less than 3 percent of this $19 billion, which the states have coming, was spent on preventing and controlling tobacco use. This is where we should be spending our money, stopping it from starting.

Remember, the whole group of lung cancers, and there are several different kinds, are among the most incurable of all the kinds of cancer we know. The diagnosis, in fact, of something called "small cell lung cancer," which is quite common and is secondary to smoking, is in itself a contraindication to surgery. We don't even offer those patients surgery because there's so little chance that surgery will help them in any way.

My personal belief is that for the moment, we do have a way to eliminate all but a very few of those more than 200,000 cases and more than the 160,000 deaths at virtually no cost at all. We just have to stop smoking, if we're smoking. Then we have to not start if we haven't started yet.

Between the American Cancer Society and other medical and governmental organizations, there's a huge abundance of resources and medical assistance to help you stop. If you're a smoker, check into those and see if you can stop smoking.

With secondhand smoke there's also a lot of controversy, but it's now pretty clear. Since secondhand smoke is now well established as a lung cancer risk, the smoker is really contributing to the development of cancer in other people. One of the rationales for preventing smoking in restaurants is really to protect not just the customers, because they can choose to vote with their wallet and go somewhere else, but it's to prevent lung cancer in the employees who work there who have no choice in their secondhand smoke exposure, and they have to work there all day. It has been an important step to make that mandatory.

In thirdhand smoke, which we defined before as the smoke residues that get into the environment, to our carpet and our upholstery and so on, this may be affecting children far greater than we know. Studies are now underway, but

I want you to try to use in your judgment a test that I think is important all through life.

You have to ask yourself which mistake would you rather make. When you're choosing between two choices like wearing a seatbelt or not, you can say to yourself, oh which mistake would I rather make? Would I rather wear my seatbelt my whole life and never have it save my life or would I rather not wear it and need it that one time? The same thing goes with exposing your children to second or thirdhand smoke and whether they should take up smoking themselves as they get older. This is our responsibility. We need to be on top of this.

Enough about smoking. I think you've heard quite probably more than you want to hear. Let's talk about blood pressure, but I'm going to come back to smoking for just a minute. Just for openers, the effects of hypertension because of smoking, high blood pressure secondary to smoking, it's something else that we can control.

Let me tell you about the physiology. Basically the tobacco products increase what we call our "sympathetic nervous system activity." This is the part of our nervous system that releases adrenalin. It's the fight, flight, fight reaction which gets your heart pumping, which gets your muscles pumping, which opens your eyes so it can emit more light. It's a survival effect. It increases the heart muscle oxygen consumption by raising the blood pressure. It increases the rate of the heart and the force of contraction. All this has downstream effects because it causes stiffening of the arteries which can last for decades. Even after you stop smoking it takes many, many, many years for that to come back to normal, but it will.

For the moment, however, while you're smoking, the reasons for your blood pressure to rise, all the chemical changes probably go up with every single cigarette you smoke. Stopping smoking can lower the risk of coronary artery heart disease by 33 percent in a relatively short period of time, even if the smoking has been going on for a long time. It's also the most significant independent factor underlying progressive kidney disease, which also leads to high blood pressure. So there are all these interlinked connections that are eventually going to get the best of you and probably kill you.

Okay this time I mean it. We're not going to talk any more about smoking.

Now let's talk about high blood pressure. This is what we call "The Silent Killer" and I mentioned it before and we need to talk about it again. What we need for all of us is very, very aggressive surveillance. In other words we need to just take people's blood pressure. It's very cheap. It's very easy. It's very accurate and it's available. You can take your own blood pressure.

They are available in the doctor's office and it's hard to go through a doctor's office without getting your blood pressure taken, but pharmacies all around the country have free machines. Many supermarkets have them today and they're reasonably inexpensive and accurate as home monitors, which you can buy and keep at home. They last forever, they require no upkeep and they're very easy to use. Most of them even remember your measurements from before.

We have lowered the limits to what is acceptable to about 120/80 as I mentioned to you and that is where we make a very sharp cutoff before we at least investigate what we want to do for the patient.

There is treatment for this. We want to have a surveillance that has treatment as we mentioned before. First of all there are life-style changes that are very, very easy and they do work. In the hypertensive patient, a decrease in salt intake can make huge differences. This may not be true for normal people. It might not make any difference at all, but if your blood pressure is already high, that may be the only thing necessary to get it back to a more acceptable level.

Exercise is the next one that is well-known to reduce blood pressure over the long term. Adopting an exercise program if you haven't had one before is very, very beneficial. Weight loss is another one, very significant factor, and then changes in nutritional choices. There is a program which I'd like you to look up on the Internet called "DASH," Dietary Approaches to Stop Hypertension. The American Heart Association has looked at this program along with the NIH and others and they have found that it is able to lower blood pressure in only a few weeks in many, many people.

We can control many of the risk factors for blood pressure. We can modify our stress level, which I will talk to you about at great length very late in the course. We have lots of good medications to get the levels down to near normal, and that's imperative for a lot of people. For those who can't get it down other ways, then we need to go on blood pressure medicine. We can treat the "bad" cholesterol, which we'll talk about, and we can use diet and statins to get our blood vessels softened up a bit so that the blood pressure will come down too.

We can reduce alcohol intake to at least a moderate amount or to zero, because undetected alcoholism is a very common finding among people with high blood pressure, something they hadn't looked at before. A very substantial payoff in reducing overall mortality and morbidity, in other words heart attacks, strokes, et cetera, will happen with these modifications and changes. This is really one where we don't have to go to Shangri-La, we can do this right in our own living rooms.

Next we're going to talk about immunizations, something very important, very dear to me. We should move on to the proactive steps that we can take to prevent disease and maintain our optimal health and immunization is right there in front of us. They have played a role for a very long time increasing life span all around the world. It started in the late 1700s.

The word "vaccination" came from "vaca" for cow. Edward Jenner in England used cow-pox, a related disease to smallpox, to immunize against smallpox. Now this was another low point in medical ethics. He did it to an 8-year-old boy who wasn't told what was happening, whose parents weren't told what was going on with this child, and he didn't know whether he could protect the child from smallpox when he exposed him to it. Fortunately for the child, and very fortunately for us, the vaccination worked, protected that child, and we have now found that smallpox is the first disease of an infectious nature that has been wiped from the face of the Earth.

We then in the '50s and '60s had the development of the Salk and the Sabin polio vaccines, which was very important to my generation, and there are lots of resources for you out there. There are about 50,000 Americans a year, mostly adults, 50,000 who die from some vaccine-preventable disease. That's an enormous number when we have the facilities and the ability to stop this. Vaccines in adults could prevent about 80 percent of all influenza deaths, about 60 percent of what we call "invasive pneumococcal disease"—this is a bacteria—and 90 percent of hepatitis deaths, because there are several kinds of hepatitis, which is inflammation of the liver usually from a virus, that can be very fatal.

Forty thousand Americans die every year from pneumococcal infections, again the bacteria, more than from any other vaccine-preventable disease. In people over 65, influenza is the most common infectious cause of death in the United States. We can do a lot to prevent that.

The big controversy comes in childhood vaccines. Still very controversial to the extent that there is a conflict that arises between the laws requiring vaccinations for admission to our public schools, a preventive health public health measure, and the parents' wishes in some cases that their children not be vaccinated, but which then presents the possibility that they could be bringing an infectious disease to school. You all should have very easy access to the latest recommendations for your children if you go to the Centers for Disease Control website, very easy to navigate, and you can get all the information you need.

It's continuously updated. It's revised information that does change on immunizations that are available. You can also go to the Advisory Committee on Immunization Practices, the American Academy of Family Physicians, the American Academy of Pediatrics, and then the Committee on Infectious Diseases, and the Centers for Disease Control and Prevention, the CDC again. They all have great websites, you can get a lot of information.

There's also a National Vaccine Immunization Program primarily for children and it's been hugely successful, tremendous gains in public health. For example, there is a disease called "invasive haemophilus influenzae type b," Hib infection. This is very prevalent among children under 5, it was the leading cause of bacterial meningitis, which is inflammation of the covering of the brains, and it caused meningitis and brain damage as well. It caused pneumonia, it caused other infections of the blood, the joints, the bones, the covering of the heart, very, very high death rate in children.

After the vaccine was introduced in 1987, the disease decreased by 99 percent in children under 5 by 2000. It was an enormous success. Again, among all the controversy, the rewards of widespread vaccination far outweigh the risks. There's no question about that. There are standard immunizations available in the United States for children. Many, many programs can be had through the government and through private agencies. Some of the controversy and concern arose over a couple of issues and one of the most important was something about mercury.

There is a preservative that was used in vaccines called "thimerosal" which contained mercury, and people felt that the thimerosal might induce mercury poisoning in their children. This came up in around 1999. The American Academy of Pediatrics and the other organizations and academies that I mentioned just suggested that the standard childhood vaccines be produced without using the mercury preservative. In the United States, since July of 2000, thimerosal-free hepatitis B vaccine, Hib vaccine, diphtheria, tetanus, and pertussis vaccine, very commonly used, have all been available to children, with no mercury.

The other vaccines, which children get – varicella, inactivated polio vaccine, and pneumococcal vaccines – all never had mercury in them to begin with. What I would recommend is that you and your family work closely with all your healthcare team, your pediatrician, your internist, your general practitioner, and perhaps infectious disease experts if necessary, to ascertain what your options are for you and your children to go ahead and follow a good plan of immunization.

There are a great many vaccines and immunizations available for the general adult population, and I want to just mention a few of them so that they're not forgotten in the shuffle. Pneumococcal vaccine which prevents a very, very deadly pneumonia in the elderly. This is a vaccine that's safe and available and can prevent a real killer in a population that has lowered resistance to it. Influenza, we have this yearly influenza, if not totally preventative it does result in a lowered severe illness. There are fewer symptoms, a much lower mortality than there might be without it, even if you get the influenza.

I happened to contract typhus while trekking in Nepal and I had the vaccine before I went. When I got home I was deathly sick. I had 107 fever, I was delirious, but I didn't die from the disease and probably because I had the vaccine. It didn't give me 100 percent protection, but it made an enormous difference.

Another one that we want to talk about is shingles vaccine. Shingles is herpes zoster, very closely related to chicken pox. If you've had chicken pox you are at risk. There is a vaccine called "Zostavax." It has been approved for people 60 years and older. It reduces the risk of shingles by approximately half, 50 percent, it doesn't give you 100 percent protection, but what we get it for is not because shingles threatens our life, but it's a very debilitating disease that can be recurrent. There's something called "post-herpetic neuralgia," meaning after the herpes virus infection you get pain in your nerves, and this reduction is about 65 percent. In a third of the untreated people over 60, the post herpetic neuralgia can become very painful and chronic.

What happens is these viruses live in your nerves after you've been cured from the chicken pox and then they tend to recur after periods of stress. This is probably a very good recommendation, it doesn't improve mortality figures, but it certainly improves morbidity.

The other vaccinations we generally know about are for things like tetanus. We have a totally preventable disease, completely safe, otherwise a severe disease with very fatal outcomes. There are other vaccines recommended for elderly people who have intercurrent disease, other diseases that might make them more susceptible. Hepatitis-A is recommended. This is carried in food and water illnesses. You can get this for example if you're a surfer who's in the water, or a swimmer off big cities after rainstorms and sewage comes into the ocean.

Hepatitis-B can be very, very severe to a very mild illness, but can also cause death, liver cancer, or cirrhosis, which is rare, but it can happen to you. Human papillomavirus which has now been linked to cancer of the uterine cervix has been recommended for its vaccine in young women to prevent cervical cancer and seems to be quite effective, although it's new and has had so far pretty good follow-up and good success.

Turning away from the vaccines, the other thing I wanted to talk to you a little bit about was dental care, which seems kind of mundane, but it's not. We happen to lead the world in good dental care at an enormous cost, but we tend to have very good teeth. There's very unequal distribution however through our population, because a lot of people have cavities, periodontal disease, tooth loss, jaw problems, and infections. The problem is that these mouth infections can cause heart disease. We can get bacteria from our mouth landing on our heart valves and this can be very serious. This can be prevented and treated. Brushing, flossing, regular preventive dental care all work right from childhood on up.

The last thing I do want to mention before we leave because it's often overlooked is hearing loss. This is a very emotionally- and psychologically-damaging problem. People who are deaf have enormous problems in keeping contact with their surroundings and their environment. They have a high incidence of depression and this is something that's very, very treatable when diagnosed. It can be prevented by preventing noise levels from reaching your ear drums when they're too high, and lots of treatment which includes surgery, hearing aids, and it is very important that you get your kids to keep proper levels of, for example, their MP3 players or even their speakers.

Chronic high levels of noise have damaging effects to the nerves within the ears and those are irreversible, and they're often not detected until it's way too late. We need to protect our children from that kind of trauma to their nerves before we detect hearing loss. Prevention is the best thing.

When we go on in our next lecture, we'll move into seeing how we can provide optimal aging all the way through our lives.

How We Look—Surgery and Skin-Care
Lecture 8

> My concern is that [cosmetic] procedures are being overly used, especially in younger patients and even in children, as one more step toward some kind of perfection which they think will meet the ideals of others and, again, in the older patient, in pursuit of this idea of eternal youth.

This lecture looks at cosmetic procedures, which are designed to improve appearance, and reconstructive procedures, which aim to improve function. Reconstructive procedures include ones you're probably familiar with, such as cleft lip and palate reconstruction. A major reconstructive procedure may also be required after removal of a cancerous tumor or as after traumatic tissue loss.

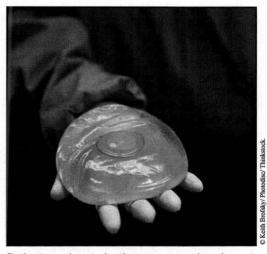

© Keith Brofsky/ Photodisc/ Thinkstock.

Patients seek out plastic surgery, such as breast implants, for cosmetic or reconstructive reasons.

Mamoplasty (reshaping of the breast) is among the most common reconstructive procedures. In augmentation mammoplasty, which is usually cosmetic, an implant is placed beneath the pectoral muscle to push out the chest wall. Reduction mammoplasty is performed for patients who have heavy breasts that cause back or neck pain. In postmastectomy reconstruction, the entire organ is reconstructed from tissues in the general area of the breast or other areas, such as the abdomen.

In 2007, 12 million cosmetic surgical procedures were performed in the United States. These included liposuction, rhinoplasty, eyelid surgery, and **abdominoplasty**. Many people who choose these treatments feel an enormous gain in self-image and confidence, but we must take care as a society not to overemphasize physical beauty and youth.

Facelifts offer excellent cosmetic results, but the procedure is not minor. Incisions are made along the face and behind the ear; the skin is then lifted up and dissected to detach it from surrounding muscle and nerves. Finally, the skin is pulled back and sewn up. The possibility exists for a high degree of blood loss in this area of the body. Rhinoplasty is another major procedure, requiring broken bones in the nose.

Botox is also a popular cosmetic option. This injectable substance comes from an organism called *Clostridium botulinum,* which produces the most deadly known toxin. Botulinum toxin acts on the neuromuscular junction, the point where nerves meet muscles, causing flaccid paralysis. Used cosmetically, it paralyzes the muscles that may have been pulling together a wrinkle, allowing the wrinkle to relax. Botox treatments have to be renewed about twice a year and are very expensive. Botox itself and artificial Botox can result in serious complications or death when the toxin migrates to other parts of the body.

Many people are concerned with cellulite, but it's important to note that there is no difference between normal fat and cellulite, and there are no medicines or creams that will magically remove cellulite. Liposuction is another popular way to remove fat, but reducing fat mass and weight in this way doesn't lower the risks associated with obesity.

The skin is our largest organ, and it may be one of the key things that drives people to plastic surgery. Exposure to the sun carries significant risks for skin damage and skin cancer. The best advice is to stay out of the sun as much as possible and use a lotion or spray with a sun protective factor (SPF) of at least 15 when you're outside. Another skin problem that affects both adults and teenagers is acne, which is basically a blocking of the sebaceous glands of the skin. Treatment may involve soap or astringents, topical drugs, and antibiotics taken by mouth. ■

abdominoplasty: Surgical removal of excess skin and fat to flatten out the abdomen.

mammoplasty: Surgical reshaping of the breast.

1. Discuss the physiology of the use of Botox for cosmetic purposes. What are the pros and cons of its use?

2. Why is proper skin care important at any age? At what age should you start taking care of your skin?

How We Look—Surgery and Skin-Care
Lecture 8

Welcome back. Today we're going to look at some of the cosmetic and plastic procedures that are available to people because how we look defines a lot about how we feel about ourselves in the context of societal norms, what people think we should look like. It's important to distinguish cosmetic procedures from reconstructive procedures.

What we mean by that is in reconstruction we're really talking about a primary aim of improving function. While the cosmetic procedures are designed to improve appearance, to bring it in line with personal and cultural norms and preferences. So that while they're generally combined, such as repair of a cleft lip and palate in a baby, we have both functional and cosmetic aspects addressed at the same time.

Some of the examples of, for example, surgical reconstructive procedures include ones you're probably familiar with. There's cleft lip and palate reconstruction and repair, which is always on a newborn baby because those babies are born with this defect. It's not acquired, and I'll talk more about that in a minute. There are things like burn scar contractions where someone may have a scar crossing a joint and it limits its contraction and it limits their ability to extend so we can release those and allow function to return. That's really not very cosmetic at all.

Sometimes we have to close big soft tissue defects after, for example, a cancer removal where lots of tissue is removed. There are major reconstructions in traumatic tissue loss, for example in big car accidents or during war. These often include the need for what we call "pedicle grafts" or "free grafts" as well. A free graft is when you take skin from one part of the body, very, very thin, thousandths of an inch thick, and put it on another. Pedicle grafts usually preserve blood supply, we may actually rotate a whole piece of skin and vessel and sometimes muscle to cover a big, deep, functioning loss.

One of the most common procedures happens to be breast procedures in reconstruction. Cosmetic augmentation mammoplasty is what it's called, "mammoplasty" just means reshaping of the breast, and in this case we usually take an implant of some kind, usually silicone, and place it beneath, not the breast but actually beneath the pectoral muscle so that the whole chest wall is pushed out, but the breast is still the tissue in front.

It tends to be very expensive surgery. It's not covered by insurance the way most of these are not covered by insurance and it's relatively a minor procedure. By that I mean there's no major body cavity that's entered or violated, the chest, the abdomen, the brain, this is all basically a big skin procedure so the risks are relatively low, but there are risks. Generally there are very, very good results and patients seem to be very happy with them.

The opposite end of this is what we call "reduction mammoplasty" and these are patients who are not generally really having the procedure for cosmetic reasons. It's usually indicated because they have breasts that are very, very heavy and often cause back pain and neck pain and actually physically get in the way of what they want to do in sports or in everyday life. It's a very significant surgical procedure because in order to reshape the breast several incisions have to be made. We can't do this through a one single hidden incision because we've got to get rid of excess skin and get breast reconstruction and molding done. The patient does have significant scarring. That's why I put it with really reconstructive surgery as opposed to cosmetic surgery.

Then there's the whole area of post-mastectomy reconstruction. These are the patients who have had the breast removed because of cancer. This is really very, very different from cosmetic breast augmentation because we're going from a situation where there is now no breast at all to try to reconstruct the entire organ from previous tissues that are there in the neighborhood and other tissues that may be moved actually from long distances like the abdomen.

There's a lot of controversy about this between people who want to do this procedure right away in the operating room at the time of the mastectomy versus those who think they should be delayed. My personal bias is heavily toward delayed reconstruction and the reason is that it's technically, in my opinion, much safer to wait, let all the surgical changes heal, because in mastectomy there's a lot of injury to blood vessels and to nerves, there's swelling, and it can be a fairly long procedure. I believe that you're compromising the possibility of a good result when you add another several hours of surgery onto an area that's already been operated on for an hour or so.

I also have a lot of other considerations that are not scientific, they just come from my experience with several thousand patients. I believe patients need time to deal with the whole idea of cancer as opposed to the idea of the cosmetics. What can happen, and I don't think it's a good thing, is patients can get so focused on the cosmetic aspect that they push aside dealing with their cancers, which to me is the primary issue in recovery and in happiness. I think the two of them can come into conflict.

Often in a lot of patients 6 or 12 months down the line, they find that life is pretty good, if they haven't had the reconstruction, and that they are still loved, that their sexuality has not been impaired, and they are healed up and they look back and think why do I want to go through another big expensive procedure when things are pretty good as they are. Many, many patients choose not to have anything done.

There's also another issue which is really again rather interesting. The patients seem to have greater satisfaction, in my observation, when they've gone from a mastectomy scar, which is pretty significant, to their reconstruction. When they go into the operating room with a normal breast and come back with a reconstructed breast, I don't think they're as happy. They are in effect trying to decide whether to wear a prosthesis underneath their bra or underneath their skin, and that's a very personal choice. They really, really don't have to make that decision right away, in my opinion. I think it's something that should wait.

Examples of cosmetic surgical procedures, these are an enormous number in our country. There are 12 million cosmetic surgical procedures which were done in 2007. Leading the pack in just big, big numbers are breast augmentation, which we talked about, liposuction, which I'm going to talk about, cosmetic rhinoplasty, which means reshaping the nose for cosmetic reasons as opposed to somebody with a deviated septum who can't breathe, eyelid surgery, and something called "abdominoplasty" which is just removing excess skin and fat to flatten out the abdomen.

There's a lot of variation in cosmetic surgery in cultures and in countries because over history there've been lots of definitions about beauty and personal identity and what is pretty and what isn't. The question of whether obesity and a lot of obesity versus thinness and real thinness has varied from country to country and from time to time so the norms are different.

Tattooing, which was when I was young very, very cultural. In this country it was usually limited, actually, to sailors who got their tattoos overseas and in other countries like New Zealand where the Māori always have had a lot of tattooing on their face and other parts of their body to now where it crosses all lines. Almost everybody in every country has different opinions about tattooing, but it's not seen as something extraordinary.

The same thing goes with piercings and enlargement of different parts of the body like the lips in Africa or the ears in other countries. They're personal choices; they have no bearing on longevity or function, which is the subject of this course, but we need to address them because people are going to be doing these procedures and we have to know about the risks and the rewards and the costs.

In our country millions of people, as I said, choose it and it costs us multiple billions of dollars. My concern is that these procedures are being overly used, especially in younger patients and even in children, as one more step towards some kind of perfection which they think will meet the ideals of others and again in the older patient in pursuit of this idea of eternal youth.

I recognize there's a positive side. Many people who choose these treatments feel an enormous gain in self-image and confidence. Many times it has changed their lives; I've seen it in my own patients and there are substantial gains in the "happiness factor." I do have to come back to my own personal concern regarding the strong correlation in our society with the over-emphasis on particular norms which define physical beauty and youth. This is not the place where we want to judge this, but I think that it is critical that we review and balance the risk and the rewards.

Let me start with facelifts because they're one of the most common procedures. If you want to know what you're going to look like with a facelift, you don't have to go to a plastic surgeon; you don't have to go to digital photography and imaging. Just go into your bathroom, close the door when nobody's around and go up to the mirror and just pull your skin back. That's what you're going to look like. Remember you've got all this skin back here that's going to have to be removed.

Having said that, in the hands of a well-trained surgeon there are excellent cosmetic results, very long periods of time, for years it's going to look good, but it's a major procedure because to do what I just said you need to make incisions along the face, sometimes behind the ear, and then lift up the skin and dissect under with either a knife or scissors to get the skin away from the underlying muscle and nerves and then pull the skin back and sew it up.

There is a lot of opportunity for bleeding because this part of the body is very well vascularized. It has lots of blood vessels, which is what makes it a place that heals well and is resistant to infection, but you can get a lot of blood loss. It may need renewal after some time, usually many years, and you have to take care of your skin. You have to avoid the recurrence of wrinkles because otherwise you'll have to be doing this again. You need to avoid the sun; of course stop smoking if you are smoking.

Problems also with some contrasts, people who have had facelifts look so good until we look at their hands or their neck, which may not have been done. It just may call attention to the facelift itself.

Let me talk to you for just a minute about rhinoplasty, another one of the very, very common procedures, and this is merely what we call a "nose job." It is a major procedure. It requires risks and expense. Bones have to be broken and there are three bones in the nose, two on the side, and one down the middle, they're often chiseled, broken, so they can be collapsed and set back. Skin may have to be removed to make the nostrils look good and under the tip so that that's all brought into proportion. This is not a small operation. You're then placed in somewhat of an external cast until your bones heal. Excellent cosmetic results. It lasts a lifetime and people are often very, very happy with this.

The other big cosmetic option that I want to talk to you about is Botox because it's so popular. Remember that this comes from an organism called *"Clostridium botulinum,"* which produces a toxin. This is the most deadly toxin in the world, bar none. Milligram for milligram there's absolutely nothing that's more poisonous than this. It acts on the neuromuscular junction, meaning where your nerve meets your muscles. There are little transmitters called "acetylcholine" that jump across and cause your muscles to contract.

When this toxin gets in there, the botulinum toxin, it causes what's called "flaccid paralysis." People who die of this toxin by eating badly-prepared food die of suffocation. Their respiratory muscles stop working. Originally it was used to cure people with crossed eyes. They would inject the toxin into the muscles to let the eyes balance; people who had uncontrolled blinking or severe nervous muscle contractions and spasms, that's how it got its start in medicine.

In 2002 though, the FDA approved Botox for cosmetic use. Five years later injections of this substance became the most-common cosmetic procedure in the U.S., about 4.5 million procedures annually. What it does is it paralyzes the muscle so that muscles that may have been, for example, pulling a wrinkle together are now paralyzed and it allows the wrinkle to be relaxed because the muscle is relaxed.

Unlike a surgical facelift it reverses itself in the body in a very few months. It's carried away from the site by the body and so it has to be renewed about twice a year. It's very expensive. It's a very toxic substance and we have had reports of serious complications when this toxin moves away to other parts of the body causing weakness or paralysis in other sites. Muscles of swallowing or respiration can be affected, very, very dangerous if it gets out of hand. There actually have been reported deaths from fake Botox preparations because profits and the enormous amount of money involved make this very appealing for people to counterfeit the drug and try to sell it.

A few words of caution: The CDC studied 1,400 adverse reactions in 2005. There were many serious results, several fatalities, and some were caused in people who were already sick, they had underlying medical problems; there was bad technique, incorrect dosage, and the danger of the drug itself. I'm talking about the counterfeit drug. Also again very expensive and it must be repeated over and over again, and now we're getting increasing concerns about bootleg Botox used by non-professionals. There are amateur Botox parties where people are buying the drug illegally, and may be getting bad drugs, and doing it themselves.

I need to talk to you now about cellulite. It sounds like a frivolous topic, but it's really not. I believe there's no such thing as cellulite. Not everybody agrees with me, but a good part of the medical community does. This term arose in about the 1920s in Europe and then it kind of drifted across the ocean here a couple of decades later.

Some people will argue the point but there is no difference between normal fat and what they call "cellulite." It's absolutely the same when you look under the microscope and you test it biologically. Those little bumps of crinkled skin that we are referring to when we say "cellulite" is due to just normal fat that has pushed up and out because there's more of it than there should be, and it's not restrained by normal connective tissue strands underneath the skin.

We see this every day. You don't need a microscope. In the operating room in surgery and in the anatomy lab you can open up the skin and see the little strands holding the fat in place. In the breasts it even has its own name; it's called "Cooper's ligaments." It keeps the fat in place. It's not free, fat is not free to glide around the body under the skin, because if it were then we would stand for a long time and find all our fat around our ankles. It doesn't happen that way. It stays in place. It's merely too much fat that becomes visible when it gets to a certain point, especially in the thighs and the abdomen.

I mention it because I don't want you to fall for the ads that are trying to sell you things to remove cellulite. This includes medicines and creams that you rub on your thighs and even surgery. Those things don't work any better than just losing the weight, and in my opinion, the cellulite-removal industry is just one enormous hoax. Don't fall for it.

Liposuction is another very, very popular way to remove fat. Since we just talked about cellulite it would be nice if it weren't contained by those septa because then you could take a suction probe, which is what they use, stick it under the skin and suck out all the fat from all over the body. Because of the containment of fat, though, the surgeon has to take the probe—and it's a sharp probe with suction on it—and force it through all the different areas, breaking down those septa, and then sucking out all the fat. It's very extensive surgery. It has definite risks. It leaves a lot of redundant skin if you've had a lot of fat removed and that skin may have to be cut out later and put back together so that you don't have a cosmetic result that's not acceptable because of now the bagginess of the skin instead of the fat.

It's important to understand that the procedures to remove fat by what we call "aspiration" can fail, because if the patient re-gains that weight, you're back exactly where you started from and then again you have more stretching of the skin, which can be more difficult to deal with. The important point is that all this reduction in fat mass and weight doesn't lower any of your risks associated with obesity.

It is not going to improve insulin sensitivity, which I'm going to talk about later, and it's not going to improve the metabolic syndrome, which is a very dangerous condition, which I'll talk to your about later in detail as well. It's not going to reduce any of the risk factors for coronary heart disease, which is associated with having what we call an "apple-shaped" body, and again we'll talk about that a lot. The concern for regression after the procedure is healed and then losing any benefit gained is a significant one; expensive again and lots of surgical complications.

Let's talk for a minute about skin protection because this is an important point. We have a lot of problems in terms of just cancer if skin is not protected, but also it's our largest organ. It's subject to a lot of problems and it may be one of the key things that drives people to plastic surgery. The important thing is to stay out of the sun as much as possible, using good sun protective factor when you're out there. This is a significant risk for skin damage, for wrinkles, for melanoma, a very serious skin cancer, and some of the non-melanoma skin cancers. Most of them are probably initiated during childhood, during sunburn episodes, and then show up as adults. Therefore, it's really important that we protect our kids early on from any sunburn.

I want you to know that stress also plays a role in some skin conditions, rashes and other forms, and it's an early sign of an over-stressed lifestyle. It'll show up on the skin in terms of even acne, and long-term stress actually has an effect on the quality of the skin in both the young and the old. We'll talk about that when we get to stress.

A little bit more on sun protection. It's probably very important that you do not tan on purpose, that you stay out of sun tanning booths, that you wear at least enough sun protection factor, about 15, and keep applying it liberally. You want to protect yourself against both ultraviolet A and B. You want to reapply it whenever you get out of the water or when you've been sweating a lot and even wear it on overcast days. Cover your skin if you can. Wear hats, don't get much more than the absolute minimum of sun every day, and especially between 10:00 am and 4:00 pm when the sun is right overhead and has its strongest concentration.

SPF factors, by the way, of greater than 15 may not give you much added benefit and they may increase certain allergic reactions if you're having those. People tend to under-apply sunscreens rather than use too much. I suggest you err on the side of a little bit too much.

Another interesting fact that came up from a study in Australia where they're right underneath the big hole in the ozone layer and they get a lot of skin cancer and sun damage, very outdoors-type people who love the beach. They did a study on people who used sunscreen daily versus people who used discretionary sunscreen, in other words there were people who just put it on all the time and people who used it when they were actually sunbathing or skiing or doing activities out in the sun. What they found was there was a 24 percent reduction in skin cancer in a very, very short period in the people who used it all the time.

Let me move now and talk about one more skin problem that probably affects as many people as any other and that's teen and adult acne. It's called "acne vulgaris," which means common or usual, not vulgar. It's the most common skin disorder in the United States and it has a serious impact upon social life and even employment. It's often unfortunately looked upon as a personal hygiene failure, which it is not. It has tremendous psychological effects, especially in teens and young people who are prone to this. It causes embarrassment and anxiety and shame and there is the risk of permanent scarring, which is going to then plague the patient for the rest of their lives.

It occurs in about 17 million Americans and about 85 percent of adolescents, and if you look at even small outbreaks, probably 100 percent of teenagers have some acne lesions during the time that they're teenagers. A significant number of patients also over 25 have either late-onset acne or persistent acne that just stayed with them after their teens.

What this disease is, is basically a plugging up of what we call "sebaceous glands." The sebaceous glands are all over your body in the skin and it's a little unit of a gland and a hair and a little muscle that stands the hair up and those glands lubricate and protect the skin. The glands can get plugged up and then you get this swelling, and they can get plugged up from oil, from greases, from dye in hair products that get on your forehead, cosmetic creams, and in fact water-based products are much less of a problem.

For treating the lesions we generally use a lot of soaps and detergents and astringents, which are drying agents and they do work. They'll get the sebum, which is the secretion, off but they don't decrease sebum production. It is constantly recurring. There's constant mechanical injury from scrubbing, so it tends to make things worse because it increases inflammation, something called "acne mechanica," mechanical acne from just the scrubbing. It's made worse by picking at it or rubbing your clothing against it like on your neck.

Listen to your mothers. Keep your hands off of your face because they can be sources of the bacteria that are causing the outbreak and making it worse.

Diet has been implicated, we really don't know a lot about that yet. Obesity itself is not a factor outside of diet. We think high sugar loads make it worse. Chocolate, which has actually always been the whipping boy of acne, is probably not a factor. Thank goodness! The role of diet is unsettled, but there's a lot of controversy around some of the products, again chocolate, peanuts, oils, cheese, none of it has been proven because this is probably a very personal reaction to the individual and it is maybe part of the quality of the food and also your own body chemistry.

Treatment can be both topical and systemic. We put on the skin topical drugs that are related to vitamin A called "retinoids." They tend to stop the progression of what we call "comedones," and those are zits, by slowing down the production of the cellular debris that plugs it up. They prevent the formation of new ones so it lessens the recurrence, but there are risks with retinol, this vitamin A group of drugs, because they can cause serious side effects on the skin, and we need to have that done under the attention of a doctor.

The other topical is called "benzoyl peroxide." It's an antibacterial agent. It loosens up the comedone and it helps get rid of some of the debris. We can then put on topical antibiotics which kill the bacterium that are in the sebaceous glands, and we can do the same thing with systemic antibiotics in more serious cases where you take the antibiotic by mouth. It gets secreted into those sebaceous glands and it reduces the inflammation. Most commonly used is tetracycline. This is the drug of choice because it has low cost, very efficient, but it has side effects too. In the end you really just need a good doctor for this one as well as basic hygiene, keeping your hands off your face.

In conclusion, there is a definite surgical role for cosmetic surgery, reconstructive surgery, and some of the ancillary treatment we use in getting the feeling of optimal health. Our primary focus, though, in these lectures is going to continue to be on prevention and healthy choices that we make day by day, that one-degree change to create absolute health and well-being. Some of the things as simple as not smoking and avoiding too much sun will markedly decrease the progress of wrinkling and things you don't like. Maybe it will reduce the need or the desire for facelifts too.

Next time we're going to move on and take a look at some of the more challenging areas for us to discuss, which may be at the root of much of our cultural and personal fears of aging and our obsession with youth. We'll spend a whole lecture talking about aging and death and dying.

The End of the Journey—Death and Dying
Lecture 9

In a lot of cultures, old age is not seen as a curse. It's looked upon as a source of great wisdom, worthy of respect, and it's a different way of seeing the wisdom and the experience of age.

Our society tends to deny the fact of death rather than preparing for it. A few days before he died, the American novelist William Saroyan supposedly said, "Everyone has got to die, but I've always believed that an exception would be made in my case." We should start by admitting that there are no exceptions. In this course, we're exploring how to live better and healthier lives, but our goal is not to avoid aging or dying. It's to live the healthiest, most energetic lives we can and age with as much grace as possible.

Even professionals in the medical community have gotten caught up in what journalist Bill Moyers called "the rescue fantasies of our health-care providers." We think we can cure everything, and we're supported in that belief by the growth of technology that allows us to perform what we once thought were miracles. Doctors refuse to acknowledge failure, and we view the deaths of our patients as exactly that, our ultimate failures.

Trying to keep a diagnosis secret from a family member robs that person of important choices about treatment and about how his or her remaining life will be spent. In the end, the patient usually jumps to the worst conclusions. And even if the prospect of death is one of those conclusions, once it's a fact, it's somehow easier to accept. Despite this, even doctors are often reluctant to be fully open with critically ill patients.

Over the past few years, some wonderful programs have sprung up in hospitals to help patients face the challenges of a cancer diagnosis, especially late-stage cancers. The new field of **psycho-oncology** blends the psychological, emotional, and spiritual aspects of a cancer diagnosis with the patient's physical care. One of the original programs in this field was

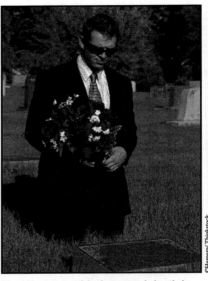

founded at Sloan-Kettering by Dr. William Breitbart, who helps patients live out their remaining time with as much fullness and awareness as possible.

Breitbart's holistic perspective on death and dying is finally being embraced in Western cultures, but it is not new to many older, more traditional cultures. I think an understanding of death grows as cultures learn to appreciate old age. Furthermore, many societies deal much more directly with death than we do. These cultures understand the cyclical nature of life and death. Death is not seen so much as the enemy but as the natural outcome of life.

Two other important developments for patients and their families who are facing death are the hospice movement and palliative care. In the hospice movement, the emphasis is on helping people die with dignity and peace. Hospice focuses on relief of symptoms and on surrounding patients with friends and family members.

The Western attidude toward death is to deny rather than prepare for it.

Palliative care is basically treatment without any intention of cure. It might include, for example, home respiratory therapy to make breathing easier for a person suffering from lung cancer. Both of these approaches have shed new light and understanding on death and dying. ■

Important Term

psycho-oncology: A medical field that combines treatment of the psychological, emotional, and spiritual aspects of coping with a cancer diagnosis with the patient's physical care.

1. Discuss some of the programs established to help patients face the diagnosis of cancer.

2. What is hospice and what services does it provide? How does it differ from palliative care?

3. Discuss your concerns or fears about aging. What steps can you take to reframe your negative ideas?

The End of the Journey—Death and Dying
Lecture 9—Transcript

Welcome back. We are probably all asking ourselves now why do we want to devote an entire lecture to death and dying in a course about optimal living and good health? It's possible that our denial of death in this culture is strongly correlated with our personal and cultural fear of aging. As we move into a lecture about death and dying, I want to say on a personal note this has unfortunately been a very timely topic for me to examine over the past year.

As someone now who is over 70, I'm watching my family and friends pass on, and for the first time I'm having to give more and more serious consideration to my own mortality. This year I lost my brother, my mother-in-law, and along with several friends, and I have other friends who are actually just teetering on the edge. This whole dance with aging and with death and longevity is a very poignant subject for me.

I think it's important that we find a way to fully embrace life long before we are threatened with death, to embrace every moment, to take nothing for granted. I've seen too many occasions where people, after receiving a life-threatening diagnosis, only then begin to do those things they had always wanted to do. We shouldn't need a scare like that to make this kind of choice. We can make the choices now, moment by moment, when we fully realize that we have a finite time, and that's a fact of life for all of us.

That's why I feel it's very important to speak to the topic with you as difficult as it may be for all of us to approach. Personally I've had my own experiences, both from a doctor's point of view, and as a member of a large and loving family. In this lecture I want to share both of those aspects with you.

I'm also learning from our culture and other cultures how to appreciate and incorporate all the various cycles into a fully-lived life. I want to quote to you from Shunryu Suzuki-Roshi, who was a very renowned Zen Master who practiced in this country for many, many years. He said, "Life is like stepping onto a boat that is about to sail out to sea and sink." Most of us don't want to address that undeniable fact until it's smack in our face.

And there's another epitaph apparently on someone's tombstone that's often quoted. It says,

> Dear stranger know as you pass by,
> As you are now, so once was I,
> As I am now, so you will be,
> Prepare yourself to follow me.

Very few of us do that. We just don't prepare. We do a very poor job, in general, of preparing for death. In our society there's practically no preparation at all, and there's lots and lots of denial. The American novelist, who some of you may know, William Saroyan, who wrote a lot about life and death, is supposed to have said a few days before he died, "Everyone has got to die, but I've always believed that an exception would be made in my case." Let's start by admitting out loud right now there are no exceptions. No one gets out of here alive.

I want to talk about some of the myths about death and dying, we don't tend to say them out loud, but in some unspoken way we're all a bit like Saroyan. There is this sense that if, the big if, we eat healthy foods and we exercise we'll be protected. We won't grow old. We will be guaranteed freedom from suffering. A good diet, exercise, that all helps, but other factors control our destiny too and we never get a 100,000 mile guarantee. You can die of melanoma skin cancer at the age of 50 that might have begun as a result of mutations that happened to you when you were a child playing at the beach in the sun.

Some people who eat the world's healthiest diets still get cancer. Some people who exercise seven days a week still die young from heart attacks. The idea is not that we'll never decline, or that we'll never become sick, and that's why we're here talking about how to live better and healthier lives. It's not to avoid aging or to avoid dying, but to live the healthiest, most energetic lives we can live and age with as much grace as possible.

We want to eat good foods. We want to create enjoyable and regular ways to move our bodies, and we want to be mindful of the whole journey. We want to make changes just because we want to feel better when we live the way the changes dictate.

On the other side of this is the current medical paradigm that's really a dilemma for me. We in the medical community have been caught up in what I believe the journalist Bill Moyers said were "the rescue fantasies of our health care providers." The rescue fantasies of our health care providers. We think we can cure everything, and we're supported in that by this burgeoning technology that allows us to do what we once thought were miracles. We absolutely refuse to acknowledge failure and we see the deaths of our patients as exactly that, our ultimate failures.

We get submerged in this fantastic medical technology that promises miracles, but in the end we're always going to lose. As the military generals say, we win many battles but ultimately, we always lose the war. In many cases, unfortunately, we actually spend more money in the last month or two of a patient's life than we had spent in the entire rest of his life combined. We struggle with even asking ourselves the hardest questions: Is the treatment worse than the disease? There was a big sign in medical school in our lounge that said, don't make the treatment worse than the disease.

Stories from our experience tend to perpetuate the myth of infallibly, we focus on those. In the 1970s my sister-in-law developed breast cancer, and at the time of her diagnosis she also had 30 out of 30 positive nodes under her arm and she had metastases to the bones of her neck. We wrote a book about this together and the title was *Never Say Die*, which tells you the attitude again that I'm talking about.

I'm not mentioning this because I want you to buy the book, don't even look for it, it's been out of print for 20 years. It's been out of date for 25 years. I just want to point out that title. She went on to have surgery, radical surgery in those days, radiation therapy, chemotherapy, and then another bout of chemotherapy. She died almost 40 years later as an older woman completely free of disease. It reinforced this whole idea that where most doctors would've said she does not have a chance to live even three years, she fooled everybody.

Then there was the 99-year-old man I told you about with the infected gallbladder in Lecture 1, and he lived to be at least 104. We remember those. As doctors we remember all our successes and we bury our failures. We perpetuate this idea that we can do anything. We also live in a society that tells us to avoid death at any cost, to keep death away until the last moment.

There are lots of old stories we tell ourselves. We say, "Don't tell daddy he has cancer..." and when we do that as a family we actually do take the choices away from the patient. When we don't tell them we put them out of the whole realm of treatment choices, of planning for whatever their remaining life is, and actually planning for death.

In my surgical practice, I happened to make a commitment early on that I was never going to talk to families away from the patients. There would be no conversations outside in the hallway. And the families would often grab me by the elbow and start to lead me out of the room and I had to say stop, and take them back to the patient's bedside. I would try to make it a habit to tell the patient in front of everybody that I'm not going to tell your family something that I'm not going to tell you, because once I do that I lose the patient's trust. Once you've lost that trust you never get it back and that's the one thing that every doctor should have between him or her and the patient.

In the end the fantasies are almost always worse for the patient than the fact. They dream of everything that could be awful. Even if the prospect of death is part of that fantasy, once it's a fact somehow it's easier to accept.

Doctors have a very hard time speaking to their patients and their patients' loved ones about dying. I think, personally, that families want honest, open discussions about prognosis so that they can prepare themselves and they can prepare the dying family member for what's ahead. Most of the doctors are reluctant to be fully open with critically-ill patients and they overstate the optimism or they just won't discuss unpleasant realities and the prognosis.

I think they believe that by holding on to hope, to give that to the patient, the patient is going to somehow have a better chance of survival. It's what doctors really believe. They're acting out of that belief, but I don't think it's necessarily true. I think that holding back critical information is very detrimental and underestimates the resiliency of the family and the patient and doesn't allow them to say goodbye or have an opportunity to say goodbye.

Now that we can, perhaps, surrender to the idea that all life does end, I want to take a look at some of the ways that are available to us so that we can help ourselves through these periods of transition. There are some new ideas in this even now, believe it or not, that can help us in this process even at this late date, big changes in our society.

Over the past few years, there've been some wonderful programs that have been springing up in hospitals to help patients face the challenges of cancer diagnosis, especially late-stage cancers, while they can still find ways to live out the rest of their lives, a length that's now been kind of spelled out for them, with meaning and with purpose. There's a whole new field and it's called "psycho-oncology," oncology meaning cancer. It blends the psychological and the emotional and the spiritual aspects of cancer and its diagnosis with the patient's physical care. It doesn't ignore that emotional side and spiritual side. The programs are now spreading through our country and actually to hospitals around the world and they've been very, very successful.

One of the original programs, which is based on what they call "Meaning Centered Therapy," Meaning Centered Therapy, was founded at the Memorial Sloan-Kettering Cancer Center in New York. They have now helped more than 300 patients in the past nine years while this has been going on, toward finding a sense of purpose and meaning while living with their cancers, especially the Stage 3 or 4 cancers, which means by definition that there's almost no chance for cure. Doctors are able to prolong life and prolong meaningful, useful life, but generally once you're in 3 or 4 you're doomed to some end probably caused by the cancer rather than something else.

The program is based on the work of the Austrian psychiatrist, who many of you have heard of, called Viktor Frankl. He himself was a survivor of the Auschwitz death camp, and he was the author of a very famous book called *Man's Search for Meaning*, which you'll find in our bibliography. Frankl wrote about the need to find "meaning." He emphasized the word "meaning" around suffering and the importance of a meaningful life as a way of coping with that suffering.

The founder of this program, a psychiatrist named Dr. William Breitbart, is helping patients live out their remaining months and years, if possible, with as much fullness and awareness as possible. It's making them mindful about this journey. There's no sense of this empty hopelessness that often surrounds the time of people waiting to die. In Breitbart's own words, he said, "Every human being wrestles with the question, how can you live knowing you're going to die?" Most of us are too distracted to think about it. Ask yourself, "What accomplishments are you most proud of? What do you want your legacy to be?" It's never, never too late.

Breitbart's patients have a whole new understanding about their dying process. Once they came to the awareness that their lives that they have lived have meaning, they examine issues such as what a meaningful death might be, what would it entail, and what would it look like. How can they face unresolved problem such as family issues before they die. They try to come to a realization that rather than dying of cancer, they are now learning to live with their disease for whatever amount of time they have. It's a very difficult road, but a very worthwhile one for them. This is similar to the sense of peace we all should seek as we all face death. It's just that for some of us, it may be without some fatal diagnosis. We're just looking forward to what we know is going to happen, we just don't know how.

Breitbart's holistic perspective on death and dying that is now finally being embraced in our Western cultures, especially here, is not new to many older, more-traditional cultures, other cultures around the world. I think an understanding of this grows as cultures find a real appreciation of old age. In a lot of cultures, old age is not seen as a curse. It's looked upon as a source of great wisdom, worthy of respect, and it's a different way of seeing the wisdom and the experience of age.

I tend to define wisdom as knowledge that has been tempered and strengthened by experience. Knowledge by itself, as we say, a little knowledge can be a dangerous thing, and it takes lots of years to temper what you know, what you've learned out of books, into real life experience. That comes with your own experience and your age and it ends up as wisdom and we can tap those sources of wisdom. Many societies prize the wisdom of their elders and elders get the respect they deserve.

Not so long, actually it is long ago, it's about 25 years now, I was in Tanzania in Africa with my wife. We were at the base of Mount Kilimanjaro waiting to climb the mountain the next day, and we went down into this tiny African village and it was a Sunday. Everybody was on their way going to church. I was walking along with my wife on a dusty path and down the road toward me came this old man who must've been in his late 80s or early 90s. He was short, very thin, and he had gnarled hands of a life of long, hard work and probably a lot of arthritis. He wore a fez, a purple fez on top of his head, and he had a double-breasted black suit on, worn and threadbare, but absolutely clean, a shirt buttoned to his neck with a white collar which was also threadbare, but clean, and he had a walking stick.

He was with a friend and he was coming toward me, and in getting ready for this trip I learned a few words of Swahili, and Swahili actually has probably the most wonderful greeting in the world. It's "Jambo," it's hard not to smile when you're saying "Jambo." "Jambo bwana," hello sir. Somebody there just had told me that in Tanzania and among Swahili-speaking people the word "mzee" means old man, but it's very, very respectful, unlike in our society where we call someone an old man it's usually pejorative. I walked down towards this man and I said, "Jambo mzee," and this man walked toward me and elbowed his friend and got a big smile on his face and he went "Mzee." He was so proud that somebody would call him old man. We need a little more of that.

On the other side of that too, similarly, a little further to the east in China, in Mandarin Chinese, which I hope I don't mutilate, the word for sir is "xiansheng" and it means "before born." What it means in detail is "you who were born before me, and therefore older, and therefore wiser, and therefore worthy of my respect." We speak again as this older person is given respect just because they're older. These are the ideas that reflect the respectful wisdom of elders, and there's much of that that we can incorporate into our own lives that's very worthwhile.

Giving respect to this wisdom that's probably there to be tapped, and then moving on in our own lives so we can be the recipient of that and deservedly be able to give our wisdom back. The same societies that have this idea – China, Tibet, much of Africa – they all deal with death much more directly than we do. There are cultures that understand the cyclical nature of life and death. Death is really not seen so much as the enemy, but the natural outcome of life. Such cultures are more often removed from miracles of modern medicine, as that village I was, in for reasons of geography or economics.

Much more of daily risk comes from just being alive. There's lots of risk around the corner. They have very strong community cultures that are tight-knit and helping each other all the time and they tend to support each other through life's transitions. We're fortunate that more and more opportunities are being created in Western culture and especially here for a community that supports patients and their family in a more inclusive and comprehensive way. Having community around you is absolutely one of the keys to a long and joyful life. We'll talk more about that as we move on and as we look back to those zones, the places where people live a long time.

We have to come back to the journey of the dying, the movement toward that moment where our life's destination is and ends. I want to just mention a bit the role of hospice and palliative care, two kind of separate entities. One of the ways we continue to create community in our culture is being able to be with people who are dying, comfortably with them, and to be with their families in a supportive way. This is where the hospice movement and palliative care have been absolutely superb. We owe a great deal to the courage of people like Elisabeth Kubler-Ross and even before her, Cicely Saunders in the de-medicalization of dying, and they have made that much, much more acceptable, taking the dying process away from the medical community as much as possible.

Hospice actually began back in medieval times. It's a very old concept. In those days it was a place, a place where travelers and the sick could just come and find rest and safety and comfort. Today, hospice basically provides care to patients and the families who are facing dying. Unlike the medieval hospice, it is a kind of care and not necessarily just a place of care. It's what they do that's important. Their emphasis is on helping people die with dignity and with peace.

They are surrounded by friends, hopefully, and family and sometimes the only friends that the patient may have might be the hospice workers. But that's important because at least there's someone and they do this in the comfort of their home, if possible. Many of us, or most of us, probably want to die at home, not in a hospital, but the reality is in the end the majority of Americans and Europeans die in a hospital often attached to machines and to monitors in a totally-dehumanizing environment.

Hospice instead focuses on the care and not the treatment. They focus on the quality of the remainder of life, the relief of symptoms. Generally, hospice is reserved for patients with terminal illness, whether it's cancer or not, although most of them are for cancer, and for a life expectancy of about six months or less. Then they have trained volunteers who relieve the family members of this constant burden of care. This is a very big burden often for the family members who are taking care of a patient at home, because they just don't get enough time to themselves.

Hospice in turn regards the process as totally normal, and it's available in hospitals as well. It doesn't mean you have to be home. If you need to be in a hospital for some reason or another you can get hospice while you're in the hospital.

What's different from palliation is that palliation defines treatment without any intention of cure. This often happens in cancer. We see this all the time. There are certain cancers that are very advanced. We know the patient is going to die of their cancer. Sooner or later that's going to come back and be the cause of their death. For example, patients on chemotherapy are often being treated with what we call "palliative intent," not curative intent. We know that what we're trying to do is create a longer disease-free interval when we can't detect cancer in the body as opposed to thinking it's really gone.

We want to make that as long as possible. We want to increase their symptom-free interval, but in the end we know they're going to die of a cancer. It's going to come back and win the war. We're going to, in our own terminology, lose that war. Although now we're trying to look at this as a normal, evitable journey.

Palliative care, for example, might include home respiratory therapy and a team to make a person's breathing easier while they may still have compromised breathing from, let's say, lung cancer or a removed lung. In hospice there are usually fewer doctors involved. They are replaced by the terminal care team and the team provides the care as opposed to treatment in the strict sense of the word. They're there just to lessen suffering, to ease pain, to ease anxiety.

Both of these are now international organizations widely spread throughout the world. They have shed a new light and understanding on death and dying that I hope more and more programs will continue to expand and help us on the journey, which is usually offered to patients in hospitals. Lots of people who don't make it to the hospital sometimes get left out of the loop.

I want to end with a short essay because we've come a long way in kind of a sad idea that we have to get a hold of. It is important for us to know that this is a journey, that we've got to enjoy every moment of the journey. If we think about the destination, we have to wake up and think that destination is our death. That's where it all ends. It's the journey that's important. I'm going to talk about this over and over again, whether we're talking about exercise or whether we're talking about nutrition or mindfulness or lifestyle. We have to be in the moment. We have to enjoy every moment of that journey until the end which is the destination.

I'm going to stop now and quote from one of our favorite and great social scientists, Woody Allen, and give you his perspective of how he thinks death should be if he had the option.

"In my next life I want to live my life backwards. You start out dead and you get that out of the way. Then you wake up in an old people's home feeling better every single day. You get kicked out for being too healthy and then go collect your pension, and then when you start to work, you get a gold watch and a party on your first day. You work for 40 years until you're young enough to enjoy your retirement. You party, you drink alcohol, and are generally promiscuous, then you are ready for high school. You then go to primary school, you become a kid, and you play. You have no responsibilities, you become a baby until you are born. And then you spend your last 9 months floating in luxurious spa-like conditions with central heating and room service on tap, larger quarters every day and then, Voila! You finish off as an orgasm. I rest my case."

Thank you. When we come back, we'll look into the future and talk about some of the prospects on the horizon for health, longevity, and well-being.

Health Advances on the Horizon
Lecture 10

FOXO3A is ... the major contender if you're going to look at a single gene for longevity. ... It could, in years ahead, lead us to some real advancement in understanding the biology of human aging.

This lecture explores some advances in medicine and science on the horizon that may affect our longevity, health, and well-being. As we've seen, both longevity and quality of life have improved markedly since the era of our grandparents. We can now stay healthier and be more productive for much longer than was ever possible in the past.

Before we look forward, it's interesting to think about a few past advances in medical science that seem commonplace today, such as polio and smallpox vaccines and penicillin. In technology, **CAT scan** and MRI equipment, which produce detailed images of organs inside the body, once seemed the stuff of science fiction. **Laparoscopic surgery** has also been revolutionary, significantly cutting hospital stays and recovery time for common procedures.

As a general surgeon, when I had the exciting experience of being there at the very beginning of laparoscopic surgery, this, too, was something out of *Fantastic Voyage*.

Currently, research into the forkhead box (*FOX*) gene family holds clinical promise for longevity. This group of genes produces proteins called transcription factors that attach to specific regions of the DNA and regulate downstream activity. These genes are also responsible for the formation of many organs and tissues in the embryo; they affect the cell cycle, DNA repair, and apoptosis; and they regulate other genes directly, including those in the cardiovascular and immune systems. The FOX proteins receive environmental stimuli and translate them into gene-expression programs that can somehow increase longevity and may even promote tumor suppression. In the laboratory, upregulation of *FOXO* genes has dramatically increased the longevity of worms and fruit flies. A related group of genes, *FOXO3A*, seems to have a positive effect on human life expectancy.

As we know, major connections have been found between chronic obesity and heart disease, adult-onset diabetes, and several cancers. One line of investigation related to obesity is the exploration of RNA interference. Inserting RNA into cells can inhibit the activity of selected genes. Researchers have been able to manipulate the genes of roundworms in such a way as to produce fat or thin specimens,

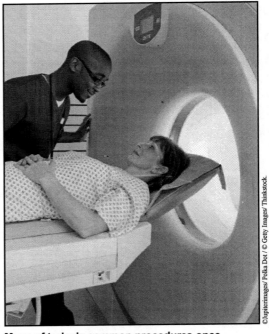

Many of today's common procedures once seemed the stuff of science fiction.

which could have implications for treating patients who have a genetic basis for obesity.

Research with primates shows that a significant reduction in calorie intake, about 30 percent, results in a marked extension of longevity, a delay in the diseases of old age, and improvement in aspects of lifestyle. However, severe calorie restriction may not work for humans for a number of reasons. For example, such diets require compulsive structuring to maintain good nutrition.

In diabetes research, work is being done to develop an artificial pancreas; this will have a computerized pump to monitor and maintain normal sugar levels in the blood. Immune retraining of the body may also help people who have **type 1 diabetes**, in which the immune system assaults the pancreatic beta cells in the islets where insulin is produced.

For patients who have **angina** and have had angioplasties, the possibilities of eluting stents are being investigated. Such stents release drugs continuously to prevent clotting. Another promising development is in biodegradable polymer technologies, which allow the delivery of doses and booster doses of vaccines in a single injection. Finally, adjuvants are additives that allow needle-free administration of vaccines, which can be particularly beneficial in trying to inoculate large numbers of children in foreign countries. ■

Important Terms

angina: Chest pain of cardiac origin caused by lack of blood flow.

CAT scan: Computerized axial tomography, a procedure used to identify disease or other abnormalities; a CAT scan machine uses computer technology to generate a three-dimensional image, or cross-section, of the body.

FOXO3A: A gene variation that appears to have a powerful positive effect on life expectancy.

laparoscopic surgery: Minimally invasive surgery using only a few small cuts into the body and an instrument through which interior structures can be seen.

type 1 diabetes: An autoimmune disorder in which the individual does not produce any insulin because the beta cells do not function; patients must take insulin throughout their lives.

1. What do you feel is the greatest medical advancement made in your lifetime? What advancement would you like to see made in the next 30 years?

2. What is the effect of severe calorie restriction (that is, a decrease of more than 30 percent of calories) on primates? Do you feel calorie restriction is a reasonable approach to lengthening life for humans?

Health Advances on the Horizon
Lecture 10—Transcript

Good day. Today, we're going to back and look at what may be out there on the horizon in the way of advances in medicine and in science that might impact our longevity, and our health and well-being. First let me go back for just a minute and review some of the good news that we covered earlier in the lectures, mainly that aging in our time, even now, has markedly improved from the era of our grandparents and our great grandparents, not only in longevity itself, the actual number of years, but more importantly in the quality of life that we might expect at the end of life.

We can now stay much healthier longer, and be more productive longer, than ever in the past. As we saw, longevity is increasing because of many, many factors. It did not include evolution, we talked about that. It included mostly advances in medicine, which was probably the biggest factor of all, nutrition, which had huge effects and I hope will have more effects on us; safety standards; and just generally more progress in healthcare, the way we eat, and standards of living.

Before we look forward from here today and into the future at what we might expect in medicine and in longevity science, I think it would be really interesting if we went back a bit and see what were some of the things that were on the horizon over the last several decades, and which now are really rather commonplace and that we take for granted. I think it will make looking forward more exciting if we can see what was once thought to be impossible and now is very much possible.

We've already talked about the advent of vaccines and newer medicines and other vaccines, for example, that treat various diseases in huge numbers. I have to remind myself how frightened our community used to be, the entire population of people in America and especially where we each lived, every summer when polio season rolled around we avoided crowds completely. We deserted the beaches in the middle of the summer. People who went to summer camps were evacuated and the kids were sent home early all because of the threat of polio. We all had friends who died in iron lungs from one of the kinds of polio that actually struck the respiratory centers at the base of the brain. We all had other friends who were paralyzed for life.

Then came the Salk and after that the Sabin oral polio vaccine in the 1950s. By the time I got to medical school, not one of us would ever actually see a case of polio again except in our textbooks. Today, there are actually only a few places in the entire world where polio exists at all. Hopefully, that too may go the way of smallpox, which was actually the first disease that was completely eradicated from the face of the Earth. It was something my grandparents and my parents could never have dreamed of, and today we take it for granted.

Even something as commonplace as the drug penicillin is really not that old. The year after I was born, penicillin was widely used for the very first time in GIs in World War II. It was so precious that it was actually recycled from the urine of those who had received it and then reused again on their wounded buddies. This led the way for a whole armada of newer and newer more powerful and widely-used antibiotics. Yet 70 years later, we have very, very little in the way of antiviral medications as opposed to antibiotics, which you know is just a bacteria.

I'm not talking about vaccines which you can use to prevent viral infections; we have lots of those. I'm talking about drugs with which we can treat viral infections once they have started. There's no viral equivalent even today of the magic bullet that penicillin was, something that selectively can kill viruses while leaving us unharmed. Penicillin does that for example to a strep throat. It will wipe out all the strep bacteria, but it doesn't hurt us at all. We're still really waiting for that one and I don't know when that's going to come. If it does and when it does come it's going to be an enormous advance. On the diagnostic side of things, some of the advances during my own career were absolutely staggering.

If you had told me when I was in medical school in the mid-1960s that one day we would have a machine that could draw like a fine pencil the entire anatomy of the body, in slices that were less than 1 cm thick, we would absolutely think you were nuts. Yet that kind of unerring detail was on the horizon just a little bit away. Ten years after I graduated, we had the first CAT scan machine, that means computerized axial tomography taking those slices. That machine was patented and very soon after that it was everywhere.

In my hospital, we bought the first CAT scan machine, we tried it out on a doctor's beagle, so we could see how it worked, and it was magic to us. That was followed by MRI, magnetic resonance imaging, which is very, very similar and it gives us pictures of organs like the brain and other parts of the body in such detail that it is absolutely astounding. To us back then, this was the stuff of science fiction. Today it's absolutely commonplace, everybody's got one. As a general surgeon, when I had the exciting experience of being there at the very beginning of laparoscopic surgery this too was something out of *Fantastic Voyage*.

In only a few months, for example, the removal of a gallbladder, which is perhaps one of the most common operations performed in America, went from a procedure that was done at very substantial risk through a big incision on the abdomen, it kept the patient in the hospital anywhere from 7 to 10 days, it required intravenous feeding for at least several of those days, very heavy doses of narcotics for pain, and a convalescent period and a stay at home of about six weeks before returning to work. Almost overnight everything changed.

When I went to learn about this we had a four-man group of surgeons and two of us went to learn the procedure and I was in a big lecture hall in Miami and there were lots of other surgeons and we had our first day's meeting and an introduction to the technique. And then the next morning we came in, the professor got up, he walked over to the microphone and he stood on the stage and he lifted up his shirt and said, "Gentlemen, this is no humbug." He had a Band-Aid here, a Band-Aid here and a Band-Aid on his navel and we all were staggered again.

We sat back and listened to him as he told us that right after the lectures he had had an attack of an acute gallbladder infection. He flew to Nashville, Tennessee, from Miami where a very famous surgeon lived, had his gallbladder out laparoscopically through the teeny TV camera through his bellybutton and two instruments that we now use to take out the gallbladder, and he was back teaching the next morning.

He said, "Gentlemen, this is no humbug." That was the statement of Dr. Warren who was the first person to operate on a patient who was asleep under anesthesia in the 1800s. He turned to the audience that was sitting around him and watching in the Massachusetts General Hospital and said, "Gentlemen, this is no humbug."

Only a year later, I was visiting the Professor of Surgery in Christ Church, New Zealand, and teaching in a hospital there and letting the surgeons in on how we do the same operations. I spent a month taking all the surgeons through the procedure and how to do it safely. By then I had done close to 400 operations. Today you routinely have this surgery as an outpatient; pain medication is very rarely required and you get back to work the next day. And yes, "This is no humbug."

What is out there on the horizon for us? Going from the look back to our now horizon and into the future. What are the stories that my medical students are going to tell their patients when they're 70 years old? This longevity research is really right up there on the frontier and I want to talk about some of the mechanisms and pathways of regulating longevity among species that are really as diverse right now as yeast, of fruit flies, worms, mice, and primates including us.

Remember, while lab experiments on other life forms don't always correlate with human experience, we do share a lot of genes with a vast variety of different animals and organisms right down to fruit flies and yeast. I suppose the fruit flies and yeast would say right down to humans. But we get good information, and we can find out a lot using these animals although many of it never comes to fruition for us, in a practical sense we get a lot out of it.

There are longevity-associated genes; we know that now. What is there on the scientific horizon that we might see to increase overall longevity? There's one mechanism with very interesting clinical promise for us. A group of proteins that are produced by a gene—that's what genes do, they produce proteins that function in our cells—and this is a gene family called "FOX." FOX stands for "Forkhead Box Family." There are 43 members of this group right now; there are probably many more we haven't discovered. I'm sure there'll be more very soon.

This whole group produces proteins called "transcription factors" which take information from DNA and moves it on to the next step. In a simple explanation, they attach to specific regions of the DNA and they regulate what we call downstream activity. One gene affects the next gene all down the line. They're responsible also for the formation of many organs and tissues in the embryo. They're very, very important genes. It's a very complicated link and it involves the turning off and turning on of these downstream genes.

However, the importance, from our point of view, is they affect cell cycle which is when cells either stay dormant in rest or turn on and reproduce. They affect DNA repair so when mistakes are made as the DNA lines up and tries to replicate itself they can be repaired, we have actual repaired genes. Then if that doesn't work they affect apoptosis, which I mentioned before, this is programmed cell suicide to get rid of defective cells and when the errors can't be corrected.

Remember the free radicals, that's our suicide pill for many of these cells. Metabolism is affected by the FOX genes. It can upregulate and downregulate energy and an important one is oxidative stress resistance. I'll talk more about that a lot later, but remember the free radicals. They create oxidative stress and we need genes to help us resist too much of it. At the end they seem to affect overall longevity.

The FOX proteins also regulate other genes directly, including those in our cardiovascular system, the heart and the vessels that supply the heart, deep down in our digestive system; a lot in the immune system, which is going to account for resistance and recovery from infections; and then cell cycle division which is not only important for new cells and building new tissues, but also for example either the development or stopping the development of cancers.

The FOX proteins receive environmental stimuli, some from the outside of our body and some that gets inside of our body and they translate them into gene expression programs that somehow can increase longevity. We don't understand how it does it just yet, and they may even promote tumor suppression. Remember I spoke about tumor suppression genes, such as the BRCA1, BRCA2, we have lots of those genes in our body that do nothing but prevent us from getting tumors, and their expression is affected one way or the other by this FOX family.

They also affect many disease states which include congenital disorders—"congenital" means with birth, so things that babies are born with. Why is this? It is because it affects things in the embryo—diabetes mellitus which occurs later on, and some cancers. In the laboratory, the upregulation of a group called "FOXO," the FOXO genes, transcription factors increase and this causes increases in lifespan which dramatically increases the longevity of worms and fruit flies.

Remember this is worms and fruit flies but we have lots of genes, including the FOX genes, which are very well conserved through evolution and they're present almost unchanged in our bodies. It's one of the things that speaks to the theory of evolution because unknown to Darwin we now can document biochemical structures that existed way, way down the life form chain all the way up to us unchanged.

Longevity in general has been affected and now by a new group in this bigger group of FOX genes called "FOXO3A," not important that you remember that. It has been shown to affect life span in worms. If the gene is switched on, then the worms live much, much longer, and if they're switched off, they don't. It's important because you can study worms that have a much shorter life span and we get a much better idea in a short period of time. If you get a 50 percent or a 75 percent increase in life, this may happen over days, weeks, or months.

In more recent studies in humans, what's really interesting is that this seems to correlate with life spans in people as well as worms and fruit flies. Investigators took samples, genetic samples, from men and women in Germany who are 100 years old or greater and what they found was the FOXO3A gene, the variation which appeared to have a powerful positive effect on human life expectancy was widely found in those people. It was found even more frequently in people that they examined that only reached 95 years of age. There's something about that gene that really gets us to the upper end of life expectancy.

In very elderly Japanese people who were also studied, there was a lot of activity of the FOXO3A genes. Remember Japan has the highest per capita number of people over 100 years old in the world. Then they returned and they did this in France, found exactly the same thing. A widely varying genetic inheritance was occurring around the world and it was not racially linked.

FOXO3A is probably now considered the major contender if you're going to look at a single gene for longevity. It's a very nice piece of science and it could in years ahead lead us to some real advancement in understanding the biology of human aging, but remember that most of these kinds of discoveries and advancements that we do in lower animals often don't come to any practical fruition in humans. Many of them die along the wayside. Some of them just don't apply and there are others that looked absolutely fabulous and then they get into human trials and something happens, they just don't work. We don't know why.

There's a lot of promise here. It'll be great to look forward to it, but it's not ready for prime time. It's a nice look ahead maybe for our children and probably more likely for our grandchildren, probably not for us to see the affects of fooling around with these genes. By the way, I always have to have reservations when we start talking about fooling around with genes. I always have that spectre of Mother Nature and the thunder and lightning and, "It's not nice to fool Mother Nature," because a lot of these do come back to bite us. It just always seems to be a two-edged sword when we get down to some of these basics.

In obesity research, another area that we're going to talk a lot about, there is a major connection between chronic obesity and heart disease, adult onset diabetes, Type II, several cancers. There's one line of investigation going on called "RNA interference." If you remember RNA is ribonucleic acid and it's a little bit like DNA, but it's one strand and it carries messages. If you insert RNA into cells, you can inhibit the activity of certain selected genes.

People took a study on roundworms, again the worms, and they have about 17,000 genes, that's not a lot. Scientists were able to find 305 of these genes and they could inhibit those genes and produce skinny little roundworms.

They took another 112 genes in the roundworm and manipulated them and they could produce fat roundworms. This has major implications for treating patients who have a strong genetic basis for obesity. For whatever the reason, at the end result, there's something in their genetic makeup which helps them remain obese even when they don't want to and try hard to lose weight, we may again very far in the future be switching genes on and off to help them.

There are some more studies on obesity, and again because obesity is such an enormous problem in our health, that may be very pertinent and you've probably read about the idea of severe calorie restriction. This ain't your regular diet. This is severe restriction. What they found is that in every organism studied from yeast to worms to fruit flies, rodents, primates, and a little bit in humans, they all show that marked reduction in calorie intake and body weight, which is about 30-33 percent, they all result in a marked extension of the length of life, a delay in the diseases of old age— those we associate with old age, arthritis and heart disease, diabetes—and improvement in aspects of lifestyle, how well people are functioning.

I'm not sure how we know what a good lifestyle is for yeast and worms and fruit flies, but we think in the primates, the monkeys that these have been tested on, they do work. We don't have a lot of information on humans yet because we have such a long life that it's going to take many, many years on people who really are on this diet, and there are not many, to see what the result is. In research at the Wisconsin Primate Institute, they took rhesus monkeys and they did show similar effects. The thinner monkeys the same age as the markedly obese monkeys had much more activity and they were much more disease-free.

The severe calorie restriction diets may not work with humans for a lot of reasons and they kind of start with Leonard Hayflick's book if you want to read that, *How and Why We Age*. Hayflick as you remember described the limit of the number of cell divisions and is quite a good expert on longevity. He pointed out some data at the Baltimore Longitudinal Study of Aging, which suggested that being very thin doesn't necessarily equate with longevity.

We don't even know if this is going to be really true with humans. The major drawback for me is practicality. It's very, very difficult for human beings to stay on this diet. A 30 percent reduction for most of us would be roughly 700 calories or more a day reduction. Most people don't like that diet. It goes against every human instinct and genetically-coded process to prevent starvation. I'm going to talk a lot about that instinct when we get to Lecture 18.

It requires major attention to the nutrients because if you're going to almost starve people, they have to have absolutely precise amounts of vitamins, of certain supplements. They have to have a balance of fat, protein, and carbohydrate that doesn't vary. They need compulsive structuring of this diet to keep it healthy because the difference between a healthy thin subject and an unhealthy starved subject is very fine, especially as we get older and we don't tolerate leeway like that too much. That's a thing we're going to have to look to and see if it's going to work.

Also, if you try to do this calorie reduction by burning more calories, in other words eating a little more but then burning more with exercise, it's not going to work out. It's going to wipe out all the gains because you're going to generate more of the damaging free radicals that can be more harmful than your benefitting from the weight loss, so we will see.

Moving on now to diabetes research, one of your great resources should be the Juvenile Diabetes Research Foundation. There is a lot of work being done on developing an artificial pancreas. In the future, still under work, it's going to try to maintain normal sugar levels in the blood as the pancreas does by having a computerized pump and having an artificial pancreas that monitors glucose continuously and regulates the pump to keep this at normal level.

There's also more on tap for Type 1 diabetes which you remember was the immune system assaulting the pancreatic beta cells in the Islets where insulin is produced. One strategy is to renew the tolerance that that patient should've had from when they were an embryo so that they don't attack their own pancreas. People recently diagnosed with Type I diabetes and who have some beta cells left might be spared losing them, so we're going to try to retrain the body with this kind of immune retraining.

There's an immune tolerance induction experiment which tries to redirect the immune system to be tolerant of the antigens that these islet cells are being seen as restoring which should've be there in the first place.

The issue of coronary artery disease is very, very complicated. Of course we're attacking this with diet and other forms of treatment to prevent it. In patients who already have coronary artery disease, we have options including stents, which we talked about; balloon angioplasty, which widens the arteries and then the stent is a metallic object or plastic that goes in to hold it open; or bypass grafts that just jump past the artery and go around it.

Patients who have angina, which is chest pain of cardiac origin from lack of blood flow, who have had angioplasties, who have widening of the coronary arteries and who have stents are all being evaluated including eluting stents, which means stents that give off drugs all the time to prevent clotting. It's a mixed bag of results and the bottom line for these patients is that whether you do angioplasty plus stent plus medication plus lifestyle changes, or you just do medications alone, it's starting to get hard to find differences in outcomes. Some of these patients do well early, some of them do well later. It's still a work in progress. We'll have to see where that goes.

One other thing I wanted to talk to you about which I think is very, very hopeful and it's going to affect a lot of people, even though it may not here in the United States, are something called "biodegradable polymer technologies." We can deliver doses and booster doses of vaccines after a single injection because like some chemicals that we take, for example enteric coated aspirin which may release in your body later, we can give people a single injection that can release again at two months and four months at six months, we don't have to wait until the patient comes back or they miss their booster dose.

The other thing that I think is absolutely wonderful is what is called "adjuvants." These are additives that allow needle-free administration of vaccines. This may not seem like a big deal, but if you remember the big thing about the polio vaccine was that fact that it could be taken orally. When you go to especially another country where there are lots of people to inoculate, just think about lining up 100 little babies in a row in their parent's arms having somebody open their mouth and then take a dropper bottle and go drop, drop, drop, drop, drop, drop and every one of those babies is going to get vaccinated by a couple of drops of vaccine in these adjuvants or in these oral vaccines.

That's so different than having to take a bottle, clean it off, open a syringe, inject it, load it up, wrestle the baby to the ground, stick him with a needle, and go on to the next baby. All this is on the horizon. It's going to revolutionize our world of infectious diseases and it's something that I just love to look ahead to.

When we come back in our next lecture we're going to start to look at a whole new topic of optimal health and well-being in regard to our nutrition. We'll look forward now at getting away from some of the genetic things that may affect us and much more into the nurture, things we can change, and we'll start with looking at the science of how our body absorbs and treats our nutritional components of our diet, and how that can improve our well-being and longevity.

Nutrition—Choices for a Healthy Life
Lecture 11

The two time-tested ways to attain optimal health without question are through healthy foods and nutrition and appropriate physical exercise or exertion. … These are going to achieve the most gain for the effort in almost all the aspects of getting to optimal health and good, healthy aging.

In the next few lectures, we'll look at general guidelines and specific suggestions for nutrition. As we do so, keep in mind our main themes for this course: moderation, the Goldilocks theory (choosing what's right for you), the idea that small changes can make a big difference, and the dictum "It's not nice to fool Mother Nature." Also remember that we will use the word "diet" in the sense of its original Greek meaning, "a way of life," rather than a weight-loss program.

In America, we're challenged by the culture of supersizing, fast foods, and an overabundance of processed foods, yet we've been saturated with false body images from the media. Our culture tends to be judgmental about people who are overweight, and we're judgmental about ourselves when we don't make our goals or manage to resculpt our images. To complicate the picture, we get mixed messages about food throughout our lives. As children, many of us were encouraged to clean our plates. Later, we're told, "Don't eat so much." In some cases, food is used as a reward or punishment. These mixed messages create mental and physical distress.

In 2006, the total cost for coronary **angioplasties** and coronary bypass operations performed in the United States was over $100 billion, but a large number of these procedures could have been avoided with basic changes in lifestyle. Furthermore, such changes can actually reverse some of the damage we've already done to ourselves. Nonetheless, some risk factors for heart disease are built into us. For example, cholesterol is introduced into the blood by two mechanisms: eating and production from the liver. The capacity of the liver to produce cholesterol is genetically determined and, in some people, may be tremendous. Today, people affected by this overproduction can take statins to block cholesterol production in the liver.

In some places, nutrition and its diseases are a matter of poverty, but in the United States, many serious diseases—including diabetes, heart disease, and cancer—can be traced to nutritional excesses. Numerous studies have shown that African, Asian, and Hispanic populations, when acquiring the diets and habits of affluent Western cultures, almost immediately begin to acquire the same diseases.

I believe there is too much focus on studying and separating out individual nutrient components in our culture instead of considering the benefit and value of the whole food. For example, a number of years ago, beta-carotene was found to be a potent antioxidant and became popular as a nutritional supplement. What people ignored, however, is the fact that there are hundreds of other carotenes in nature. Why isolate one chemical or one antioxidant property, when we can get them all by eating the whole food? Our goal is to try to find combinations that provide optimum nutrition.

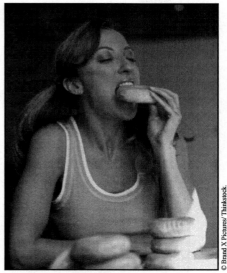

Nutrition-related disease may be linked to scarcity or to overabundance.

There are many weight-loss diets with gross nutritional imbalances. No-fat diets, for example, make it hard to absorb fat-soluble vitamins and ignore the importance of healthy fats. Low-carb or no-carb diets simulate diabetes. The key is to find nutritional balance. In the next few lectures, we'll talk about the value of cooking at home, reducing the percentage of meat in your diet, and increasing fish, fruits, grains, and vegetables. ∎

angioplasty: A medical procedure performed to widen existing coronary arteries.

Questions to Consider

1. Discuss the differences between diseases of poverty and diseases of affluence.

2. What is meant by the term "nutritional balance"? Discuss what this means to you personally in the context of the Goldilocks criteria.

Nutrition—Choices for a Healthy Life
Lecture 11—Transcript

Welcome back again. Today we're going to move into what I hope will be a very interesting series of discussions about the selections of food, about vitamins and supplements, and what we can do and choose in the form of optimal health and well-being in our pursuit of a good healthy old age.

In the next nine lectures on nutrition we'll look at general guidelines as well as some very specific suggestions for you. I want you to keep in mind along the way are key themes that are going to pervade the whole course. Moderation, again our bodies like to stay in the middle and not stray too far; our Goldilocks theory, which is going to allow us to do the choosing so that we can decide what we're going to enjoy and make it sustainable; the one degree of change in our course, no crash diets or big reversals of what we're doing; and always, not trying to fool Mother Nature.

We're going to examine goals and guidelines for good nutrition all through our various ages as we get older and the stages of our life span, and we're going to see how food choices can benefit us or harm us each as individuals. Then we'll see how the same choices can benefit or harm society as a whole, because what we choose can have effects on others and on our planet. And we'll see how the choices will affect or harm the environment generally and specifically in our own regions.

We'll make an important distinction in this series in the word "diet." I don't want to use the word "diet" whenever possible to mean how to lose weight. That's the one definition that I want to move away from when I can. We want to go back to the origin of the word in English, which comes from the Greek *diaita* 'a way of life.' I want this meaning for us to be the entire basis of our personal nutrition needs as opposed to a diet as a way to achieve specific things such as weight loss, and other things as well. This is going to become our way of life. For our own purposes, we'll just go back to the original meaning.

We'll look at the contribution of nutritional changes, whether they're very small ones or not, the one-degree change and how it helps us to get to where we want to be, especially in comparison with some of the other ways we try to strive to improve our lives. The two time-tested ways to attain optimal health without question are through healthy foods and nutrition and appropriate physical exercise, for exertion. I'd like to move away from exercise and make it more exertion, recreation, body movement. These are going to achieve the most gain for the effort in almost all the aspects of getting to optimal health and good, healthy aging.

It'll help us also maintain our mental acuity and health and provide optimal protection and prevention from serious illness. We'll maintain our overall body function and we'll feel good about it so we can enjoy our longevity. At the same time, we do have to recognize that we live in a world that challenges us with this culture of supersizing, of fast foods, and this overabundance of processed foods, which I'm going to discuss in depth throughout the series.

How many people have not been to a movie theater where somebody didn't offer you an enormous soda for 25 cents more or a freight car full of popcorn that you and your family can eat for the rest of your lives for another dime. This is always being pushed in our face. We're always having to resist, and in fact, they look at us as if we're crazy when we don't accept it. Look at the fast food movement in America, the fast food restaurants, and compare this with the whole new slow movement. We're going to look at globalization about how we have been exporting our bad habits, especially fast food and processed foods around the world.

I was brought up in Brooklyn and I lived in a family that just loved butter and well- marbled steaks and lots of red meat and saturated fats. I hate to admit it, but as I grew up, in the morning even when I was little, making my own breakfast of chocolate cupcakes and chocolate milk, and it has taken me an absolute lifetime trying to get over my sweet tooth and get that under control. I have my own issues about belly fat, and the journey to correct it is still ongoing, something many, many of us have going for us or against us.

I have a friend, a very close friend in surgery, who struggled for decades trying to get to what he thought was an optimum weight. I'm pretty sure that he tried all the various fad diets and I think that he must have lost at least a thousand pounds during his life. He had tried them all, and he finally said to me you know what, "They don't make you live longer, they just make it feel longer." And I think he's right. I think there's very little evidence that these fad diets do anything but stress you and make you more concerned about what you're eating than you should be.

This same guy by the way, while he was trying to lose some weight, I discovered Lean Cuisine when they first came out and I had one and it tasted OK to me, so I mentioned it to him. The next day we were getting ready for surgery and I said, "Well, how did you like that stuff you bought last night?" He said, "It was delicious. I had four of them." Some habits are hard to break. There are some things that just follow us around and make this path rather difficult.

In our contemporary Western culture, we've been saturated with an abundance of false images and goals that we have taken as the standards. From early in our lives, even as children, we are inundated with pictures and descriptions of how we should look, how we should feel, based on the standards of a youth-obsessed culture. We tend to look toward Hollywood and our favorite actors and actresses who are thin and they're muscular and they're sculpted and they are really gorgeous beyond reality. We forget that they spend their entire life doing this because that's the way they make their living.

Our culture creates a lot of judgment, too, around people who are overweight, who are way too often unfairly characterized as being weak or somehow "less than," that they are weak-willed or they lack discipline. We cast a shadow of shame on people who don't live up to the ideal pictures of other cultures that we have created and we have established as the norm. Worse yet, we do it to ourselves in the form of self-judgment and heaping shame upon ourselves when we don't make our goals or our images.

We make the picture even more complicated. In many of our histories I think we all remember the "Clean Plate Club." We were rewarded for cleaning our plate and not leaving anything over, so that standard became part of our psyche at a very, very early age. We were reminded, at least when I was growing up right during and after World War II, of the starving children in Hungary, or later in Armenia, or somewhere in China, and it made us even more guilty. Although I used to think and I never said it to my parents, well how am I going to help anybody in China or Hungary if I don't clean my plate. They're not going to get anymore food, and I wouldn't dare say that out loud back then.

I also remember thinking that the name of the country Hungary came because everybody there was hungry. This really must have been a big issue when I was growing up. There was this eat more, eat, eat and then later on eat less, you're eating too much. You're getting obese. The message was eat it because it's good for you, or don't eat this because it's bad for you. Then worse, eat this because it'll make you feel a lot better, or using food as a reward or as a punishment, which is a terrible thing to do.

I strongly urge everyone not to do that to their children. These messages absolutely make us nuts! They create mental and physical dis-ease. It's a no-win situation and it's crazy-making. It's insidious, it's wide spread, it crosses absolutely all generational, economic, gender, and racial lines. It goes on everywhere. Finding the correct balance in nutrition, however, is worth the effort because it's going to pay dividends way, way down the line, and you will receive far more benefit than you can imagine if we can get away from all of that.

The first thing I want to do is take one more look at surgical options open to people with coronary artery disease. I'm not going back but I want to talk to you about the usefulness and then compare it with what we should be doing in our lives instead. It's very pertinent to diet choices as you'll see in a minute. If we look at the costs either as an individual or a society, it's a very grim picture. In 2006 the American Heart Association found that there were 1.3 million coronary angioplasty procedures done in America at nearly $50,000 each, for a total U.S. bill of $60 billion. Nearly 450,000 coronary bypass operations were done, at about $100,000 each, again for a total of about $45 billion. That's over $100 billion a year for just those two operations.

In 2007 The New England Journal of Medicine produced some studies showing that angioplasties and stents may not extend life in a lot of these patients, and that coronary artery bypass surgery may prolong life in a few of them. This means we also need to assess the value of these procedures on the patient's future quality of life, considering the possibility of life as a coronary cripple, being kept in your chair or your house unable to participate in activities.

A large number of the procedures could've been avoided by basic changes in lifestyles, even if there's a strong family genetic propensity toward the disease. If we begin with good nutrition early in our childhood and maintain that, that one-degree change, we can avoid a lot of these procedures. As we look forward, before these become surgical choices for us, we should consider the results.

In a comparison of the possible future cost of hundreds of millions of dollars and considerable surgical risk and terrible pain—these are awfully big operations, especially coronary bypass where your sternum is split and then wired together—against the possibility of now, right this minute, making new personalized choices in diet and lifestyle, which we know is going to work. These changes can actually reverse some of the damage we've already done, not just stop them from progressing.

There are a lot of risk factors that are built into us, they're not choices. For example the way cholesterol is handled. That's a really big one and it makes a good example. You get cholesterol into your blood which then goes into your vessels and your liver and other places by two mechanisms. First there's the cholesterol you eat, and what you're taking in your diet is then absorbed and circulated and processed. Then there's your liver. Your liver can make cholesterol from almost anything. Give it some shoelaces, it'll break it down and make it into cholesterol. It has a tremendous capacity to do that and that is genetically determined.

In my experience, when I grew up and I was in my 40s, I discovered my cholesterol was way over the top of normal, just like many people in my family. I tried to bring it down, I dieted and dieted, cut fats and meat out of my diet, and it didn't budge. I then became a vegetarian for six years, had no animal fat, no fish fat, which by the way may be good for you—didn't know that then—and it still didn't budge. It was very clear that this was my liver producing all of the cholesterol, and diet wasn't going to matter at all.

I'm very grateful for the discovery of statins which is a drug which affects the liver production. It blocks cholesterol production in the liver, and my cholesterol just came bang down right to where it should be. There's a very reasonable chance that I might not have lived to where I am now had I not changed that part of my biology. We've got to look at both aspects. However, if we can make small changes in lifestyle, again one degree, we may be able to expand all the choices, and the surgical options may be put far in the background.

Nutritional diseases and their comparisons are really very important. The choices we make often reflect the reality of our exposure to disease. In the world there are huge differences regarding disease that comes from imbalances in nutrition. For example, in some places, nutrition and its diseases are a matter of poverty, a matter of a lack of enough nutrition. There's too little access to healthy foods and pure water. Infectious diseases then follow, such as diarrhea which kills literally millions of children every year around the world, as well as susceptibility to pneumonia, to tuberculosis, even to measles. It's mainly due to poor nutrition, that side of the scale, poor sanitation, impure water. At the other end, and maybe almost as deadly, are diseases of affluence, of abundance, and that's where we tend to be. Too much access in our case to processed foods and what we call cheap calories. We can buy calories in this country from just nothing compared to other parts of the world.

Those diseases, instead of the starvation diseases, include diabetes, very deadly; coronary artery heart disease, very deadly; obesity, we'll talk a lot about that; and then cancers, which are related to certain kinds of obese conditions including liver cancer, rectal cancer, colon cancer, lung cancer, breast cancer, stomach, esophagus; and also we have diseases of affluence that you would never think of, forgetting nutrition.

Polio in the '50s was an interesting case that wasn't related to food, but rather too little exposure to what doctors used to jokingly call vitamin D, or dirt. What happened was that polio was a disease that was fairly well tolerated by infants. They'd get sick, but they'd get over it. They didn't get paralyzed very often, and then they were immune. They could pass their immunity on to other infants and children in the family because they had the virus in their feces, and polio is passed along by the oral/fecal route. What happened in wealthier families, they were very meticulously clean. The children were washed and scrubbed and protected from dirt, from the vitamin D, and it was tending to be a disease of the wealthy rather than the poor in the United States at one time.

Going back to this, the summary is that many of the diseases in the U.S., especially nutritional, are diseases of nutritional excesses. The historical connotations, and this is recent history, of meat and fat consumption has been as a sign of affluence. In my parents' home it was absolutely the case. They were children of the Great Depression and they associated meat and fat and butter in large amounts with affluence, even though they weren't particularly rich. It was something they could put out to the world. In our home we ate meat almost every night. We ate gobs of butter on our potatoes and on our bread, and we had that whole affluent side of bad eating habits.

There is an association of Western diseases with, for example elevated blood cholesterol. This all goes together as one big package of danger. There've been lots of studies that show that African, Asian, Hispanic populations, when acquiring the diets and habits of affluent Western cultures—in other words when they immigrate here and they start adopting our diets—they almost immediately begin to acquire the same diseases.

The same was true, for example, of Japanese women who migrated to the United States. They adapted, or adopted, our culture, our environment, and our diets and they began to increase their incidence of breast cancer to levels that had been low and now were reaching that of the American native. That happened in the very generation that migrated. It happened again to Aboriginal people in Australia when they moved to the big cities. This was a very healthy group of people who then got diabetes, heart disease, obesity, strokes, all of it.

The approach to nutrition in this course is going to look at our contemporary Western cultures where I believe there is just too much focus on studying and separating out individual nutrient components—vitamins, supplements, other chemicals—instead of considering the benefit and the value of the whole food itself. We have a habit of looking at what's missing in our foods and then we try to artificially replace it, or even escalate it, so if we think a little is good, a lot must be better, and take mega doses. I think this is a very, very dangerous approach and one we have to move away from. That's one of our course corrections that's going to be moving away from something instead of toward it.

I want to in general focus on moving toward health ideas, but this is one time we're going to have to move away. We're going to focus on the value of whole food and that's going to be our goal, combinations that provide optimum nutrition. Let me give you an example of what I was just talking about. A number of years ago there was a huge popularity of beta carotene. This was a component of many, many foods like carrots and found to be a very potent antioxidant. People thought that's wonderful, let's take it out of the carrots and manufacture it if we can, put it in a pill, extract it, make it available in the synthetic form, and take lots of it.

What these scientists and promoters forgot was that there are hundreds of other carotenes in nature. In our food there are probably at least 60 of them including alpha carotene, beta carotene, gamma, delta, and so on, that may act in concert with the beta carotene and give a synergistic effect. We don't understand that very well, but nature has put those together in these foods, not for our benefit, but for the benefit of the food, and here we are separating them out. Why isolate one chemical, or one anti-oxidant property, when we can get them all by eating the whole food? We're going to learn more about that later in an example about just where this can go especially with beta carotene.

I have friends who live nearby me, a lovely family, who love juicing. Remember not the juicing of an orange that you may squeeze in the morning, but the kind of $300 juicers where you stuck in tons of carrots and the little sharp blades would extract the juice and you were left with a glass of juice and a big pile of carrot shreds on the side. These people came by one day with all the kids beaming, three little boys and the parents, and they held up their hands to me and they said look, and they had turned orange from all the carotene. Fortunately that's not dangerous in this case. They thought this was terrific. I thought this was just awful.

It was clearly showing that the body couldn't handle this much carotene, that this was a huge course change. It was not moderation. Let me just stick in my view on juicing in general. I know people love this. I know every health store in the world still sells juicers and you can still go in and have things juiced for you. It just seems to me to be extreme and you're losing a lot of the benefit in the whole food. For example, when you just get the juice you're throwing away all the fiber that's left over on the other side of that juicer and not getting any of it. There's also a lot of pleasure to be had from whole foods.

You may like juice, that's fine, go ahead and do it, but don't forget you're losing a big part of this nutrition. Also with the focus on the parts of foods' nutritional benefit, we're going to miss an important value which we get from the whole food and that's the combinations, the proportions, and the dosages of the vitamins in the food. Proper absorption, the synergy, and bioavailability, means what you can absorb, is very much part of the construction of food when we eat it as opposed to taking things out of it.

Early research in the field of nutrition has been focused basically on a limited number of nutrients. That's where it all came from in the last century, instead of whole foods. We want to go back and expand what we have learned, going from that micro-focus and expanding it up into a macro-perspective and consider the ways of eating which have been found to be of great value in preserving and maintaining health, such as variations on things like the Mediterranean diet, which I'm going to talk about at great length, which has now very much come into interest because there's a lot of science around the value of diets like that. I'll talk about it in great detail.

There are lots of diets out there with huge gross nutritional imbalances and I must admit I'm totally against them. We have low-fat or no-fat diets. No-fat diets, for example, make it hard to absorb fat-soluble vitamins. Things dissolve in like things. Water-soluble products need water. Fats need fat-soluble solutions to make them absorbable. We also forget about the importance of healthy fats, and we'll spend a lot of time on which they are and where you can get them into your diet.

There's the low-carb and the no-carb diets. The example are these diets which basically, by giving you low carbohydrate or no carbohydrate, they're absolutely simulating diabetes. The body need carbohydrate to light the fire of our metabolic cycles, which I'll tell you more about soon, and you will absolutely burn more fat, but you'll become like a diabetic, and that's not good. We'll go into the details of the chemistry later, but that was just one example of the extreme. I really don't believe in any of the extreme diets for long term. They can be very, very dangerous and I don't see the advantage of so-called "jump starting" your diet.

We need to find nutritional balance. A number of authors and experts in the field of nutrition and longevity are now speaking to the value of obtaining our nutritional needs by eating whole foods. There's a growing movement of experts, of scientists, and people who are just interested in nutrition who want to get us back to whole foods. That's where I want to place our focus because I absolutely agree 100 percent.

Those cultures which we looked at, the longest-living cultures where people attain a healthy longevity, are eating exactly what these authors are suggesting. We've put a few of our top choices in the bibliography, and I hope you'll take a good look at those when you're done listening to the course. They will all speak to the value of knowing, as best as you can, what your food is, what's in it, and what the sources are.

Getting to know your farmer or your fisherman is a bumper sticker where I live, "Who's your fisherman?" It's not easy in many places. As we move forward I'm going to have some concrete suggestions as to how you might make this happen even if your source of food is a mega-supermarket in the middle of a huge city. We'll talk a little bit of the value of cooking at home, which has the benefit of careful selection of ingredients. You will go into control of all the ingredients and you won't have to worry about what's in there.

We'll also speak to the importance of generally reducing the percentage of meat in your diet and increasing fish, fruits, grains, and vegetables. The benefits for both you and the environment are very important. Decreasing your exposure to chemicals present in most meats, decreasing dietary saturated fat and cholesterol, meat consumption in the U.S. is way, way over the healthy limits. The average American eats about a half a pound of meat a day, and we are both producing and eating a disproportionate amount of the world's meat supply.

We can do a great deal for our health as well as the environment's health by shifting proportions on our plates from meat to grains and veggies. Outside of our own personal moral considerations, I'm not suggesting that it's necessary to become a vegetarian or a vegan, but even small changes in proportion can make a major change for the good in our bodies and in the planet.

Fish is another issue. In the longest-lived cultures on earth, and in the current scientific understanding of the benefits of whole food, adding more fish in our diets is just as important. We can obtain healthy proteins that are lower in bad fat, too, and higher in good fat when we substitute fish for meat. It's also important to realize that even though fish populations have been widely depleted in recent decades, there are many viable forms of fish from sustainable and healthy sources. Farm-raised fish in most cases are not what I favor. I don't think they're the answer. They tend to have more chemicals and antibiotics polluting the fish you eat and also then getting out into the environment.

Fruits and vegetables and grains are without a doubt an important part of a healthy diet. Increasing that proportion should be a major part of your goal and has been a part of the diet of the longest-lived cultures as long as we know. Again it's the quality, the quantity, and knowing the source, one-degree changes and, of course, Goldilocks. What's going to taste good to you. There are a few vegetables that I just can't learn to like and I know they'd probably be good to me, but I just find others. There are some great ideas for finding high-quality produce. You can grow and consume at least some locally-produced produce for yourself. It's not 100 percent possible for most people, but it's a good place to start. We'll discuss all this much later.

In the following lectures, we'll begin to assemble a structure to guide you through optimal nutrition, a guide on how to avoid the fads and the unproven, and a way for you to personalize and assemble the building blocks for lifelong, solid eating habits.

The Physiology of Nutrition
Lecture 12

> In energy production ... the final common denominator is almost always glucose. It's the most familiar carbohydrate, for example, and the diet which brings us [this consists of] breads, pastas, rice, beans, and a lot of the grains.

In this lecture, we learn how our bodies process foods and nutrients in foods. The key word here is "metabolism," which refers to all the energy processes in the body, including consumption, expenditure, and renewal. Metabolism can be divided into two processes: **catabolic reactions**, which break down molecules and release energy for use by the cells, and **anabolic reactions**, which consume energy and resynthesize cells or tissues.

These energy transfers rely on a common currency in our cells, a chemical called adenosine. This is a large molecule that has two or three phosphate radicals (ADP with two phosphate radicals; ATP with three). When the adenosine has three phosphate radicals, it can release energy by releasing one of the phosphates. Conversely, energy is required to convert the resulting ADP back into ATP.

There are seven major classes of nutrients, divided into two groups. The macronutrients are required by our bodies in large amounts. These are carbohydrates, fats, proteins, fiber, and water. The micronutrients—vitamins and minerals—are required in small amounts

Carbohydrates are organic molecules made up of long chains of carbon, along with hydrogen and oxygen. Common carbohydrates are broken down into two categories: simple and complex. Simple carbohydrates, such as glucose, are absorbed rapidly by the body. In body cells that require immediate energy, glucose is oxidized and burned to produce energy via the ATP and ADP + P pathway. Excess glucose can be stored in the liver and the muscles for future use as a molecule called glycogen. To get the glucose into the cell to work, we use the hormone insulin, which comes from the islet cells of the pancreas and drives the glucose out of the blood and into the cell where it can be used.

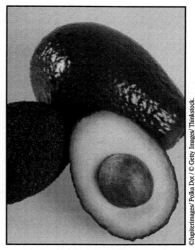

Avocados contain healthy unsaturated fats.

Most of the fats in the body are triglycerides, which are made up of a backbone molecule called glycerol with three fatty acids attached. Transportation of fats in the body is performed by lipoproteins, which also carry cholesterol. Lipoproteins are arranged into groups by their physical density. **LDL** and very low–density lipoprotein (VLDL) are mainly in the body to transport the triglycerides from liver cells to fat cells, where they're stored. LDL delivers cholesterol to cells throughout the body for tissue repair, but excessive LDL can result in fatty plaque. HDL carries excess cholesterol to the liver for destruction to prevent its accumulation in the bloodstream.

The fats we eat are classified as saturated or unsaturated. Saturated fats and trans-fats, which are the worst for your health, are generally solid at room temperature, such as butter. Unsaturated fats tend to be liquid at room temperature and are healthy, particularly monounsaturated fats. These can be found in avocado, canola oil, and olive oil.

Proteins are basically made of chains of amino acids and are used in transportation and structural functions. The essential amino acids are those we cannot make in our bodies; we have to eat them. Fortunately, we can get all we need by eating plants or other animals that have eaten plants.

Any healthy diet includes low amounts of saturated fats, lots of fruits and vegetables, and lots of whole grains, and it's generally low in sugars, cholesterol, and salt. ■

anabolic reactions: Reactions that consume energy and are used to resynthesize compounds.

catabolic reactions: Metabolic reactions that break down molecules.

LDL: Low-density lipoprotein, fat protein that transports triglycerides from liver cells to fat cells, where they are stored; carries cholesterol in the blood and delivers it to cells throughout the body for tissue repair; and aids in the synthesis of vital chemicals, such as steroid hormones.

Questions to Consider

1. Discuss in as much detail as you can the conversion of ATP to ADP plus energy.

2. Discuss the functional and physiologic differences among HDL, LDL, and total cholesterol. Do you know your own LDL and HDL levels?

The Physiology of Nutrition
Lecture 12—Transcript

Welcome back. Today, we're going to take a look at how our bodies process foods and the nutrients in those foods. The word for today is really all about metabolism. "Metabolism" refers to all the energy processes that are in our body, both of consumption and expenditure of energy, as well as renewing energy. It comes in two kinds, two flavors. There is catabolism, or catabolic reactions, and these are the reactions that break down molecules. They decompose substances, and in the processes they release energy for use by the cells. The other one of those is anabolism, or anabolic reactions, and they consume energy and are used to re-synthesize, to put things back together and rejuvenate cells or new tissues. Or they can also be used to store energy for later use and then catabolism again.

Anabolic reactions use the energy to move muscles, to do work, to think, and to consume the energy that's been released by the catabolism. It's one enormous continuous cycle of chemistry and it always has to be balanced perfectly. All the energy transfers always come down to a common currency in our cells. It's a chemical called "adenosine" and this is a very large molecule that has two or three phosphate radicals. That's phosphorous with several oxygen atoms attached, and they move together. They are attached to the adenosine, either three of those radicals called "ATP," adenosine triphosphate, and "ADP," adenosine diphosphate.

When the adenosine has all three, it's loaded and it's ready to release energy. It's like a ball at the top of a hill with potential energy to roll down. It does so when one of the phosphates is released, that's how the energy is released, and it's leaving over ADP, now only two phosphates, and the free phosphate radical out here in the environment. Conversely it takes energy to put that phosphate back on the ADP to make ATP again. It's like pushing the ball back up the hill and loading it up getting ready for another ride down.

The body uses this cycle in two main ways, fairly complicated, but always getting back to the same basics. One kind allows the ADP and the ATP cycle to go on for hours and hours. We use this for example in running a marathon. It's aerobic; it uses oxygen. There is another kind which happens where we deplete the reservoir in minutes, sometimes even seconds, of tremendous exertion as if running let's say in a very fast hundred yard dash or a 440, something that uses tremendous amounts of reserves in a short period of time. It's going to be very important that we understand this as we move ahead and explore how we utilize our sources of energy, especially later when we get into exercise and how we move our bodies.

We're going to talk a little bit about nutrients today, which is where all the energy comes from. There are seven major classes and we're going to talk about three of them today. They are divided into the macronutrients, which are required by our body in large amounts. That's why they're called "macro," it means big, and that keeps us functioning. The three we're going to talk about are carbohydrates, fats, and proteins, and we'll save the other macronutrients, fiber and water, for later.

Then there are the micronutrients, which are only required in very small amounts, sometimes what we call "trace elements" because they're barely needed in any quantity, but they're also very critical. They keep the body functioning. They include minerals, vitamins, which I'll talk about later also. We require all of them in our diet in various amounts and in varying forms. They are important to us and we have to get them from the outside. These are the fuel.

Right now we'll focus on the Big 3. We'll start with carbohydrates, and just before we get into that let me just define "organic" because that comes up in chemistry and it comes up later as choices for foods. Organic refers to biologic systems. In chemistry we're talking about the chemicals, the molecules, the atoms that are part of living biological systems, be they plants or animals high or low on the scale. It's our biology and it also happens to be based in carbon.

All the organic molecules must have a carbon base. We'll start off with carbohydrates and this is an organic molecule. It is made up of lots of carbon, often in long chains, and carbon happens to have four places where other atoms can attach. It can have one, two, three, or four of those places used up by other atoms. It also always has to have hydrogen and oxygen, and the reason it's called a "carbohydrate" is the hydrogen and oxygen is always present in the ratio that it is in water. It's two hydrogens for one oxygen, H_2O.

In common carbohydrates we want to look at another division and this breaks them down into what we call the "simple" ones, the monosaccharides. These are sugars that have only one sugar in them; glucose, which is our primary sugar and then fructose, which comes from food; galactose that comes from milk. Remember "o-s-e" means sugar. Then there are the disaccharides, meaning two of them attached together. The one you know is that sugar that's on our table called "sucrose," and it's one molecule of glucose attached to a another molecule of fructose.

Then there are the complex polysaccharides, meaning many sugars, and we know that mostly as starch. They're all very closely related and they are inter-exchangeable and rebuildable within the body. The body can get whatever it needs from these substrates and make new ones.

In energy production, however, the final common denominator is almost always glucose. It's the most familiar carbohydrate, for example, and the diet which brings us these are breads, pastas, rice, beans, and a lot of the grains. The polysaccharides are often also called "complex carbohydrates" and they take longer to digest because we've got all these molecules put together of the various sugars and they have to be broken apart and chemically snipped off from the longer chain to get to small individual molecules that we can use.

Conversely, simple carbohydrates like glucose are absorbed very, very rapidly. Blood-sugar levels can spike when they're needed, and so let's say an emergency when you need a lot of glucose, but also it's a two-edged sword because it can actually be more detrimental than beneficial. We'll look at this in great detail when we talk about why these quick rises and falls in blood sugar can lead to imbalances and even in some case disease, but that's the emergency source of the glucose.

There are several glucose pathways for using the sugar that we have and that we need. Just as an aside, our brain happens to be one of the places in the body that has absolutely no extra storage for glucose. This means that if we cut off the blood supply to the brain which is carrying glucose and oxygen to the brain, the brain will shut down in minutes. It has no reserves. In body cells that require immediate energy, other than the brain, glucose is oxidized and burned to produce energy via ATP and ADP+P as the pathway we talked about before.

Excess glucose can be stored in the liver and in the muscles for future use like emergencies as a molecule we call "glycogen." "Gen" referring to generation because it generates glucose. It must enter body cells to work. We can't use it in between cells. It has to be working right in the middle of the cell, almost always in the mitochondria, that little organelle that all our cells have and those are the engines and we feed those engines with the fuel of glucose. To get the glucose into the cell we use the hormone insulin, that comes from the Islet cells of the pancreas and drives the sugar, the glucose, out of the blood and into the cell where it can be used.

A phrase you'll hear is the "Krebs Cycle." This is a very, very complicated cycle. It is fundamentally our energy-producing cycle in the body. It is aerobic and requires oxygen to burn our fuel, and ATP is what is used to generate energy. The byproduct coming out our exhaust tanks are CO_2, carbon dioxide, and water. We know that when we exhale that's what's in a lot of our breath. We get rid of our CO_2 and some water vapor as well. Those are the byproducts of combustion.

That's so much for carbohydrates. The next group I want to talk to you about is lipid. "Lipid" means fat and we want to talk about lipid metabolism, burning and storage. These are also organic molecules naturally because they're in biologic systems and most of the fats in the body are what we call "triglycerides." These are made up of a backbone of a molecule called "glycerol," which is technically an organic alcohol, and then it has three fatty acids coming off the glycerol carbons like the capital letter "E."

Fat molecules are what are called "hydrophobic molecules." These are very important. This means they don't dissolve in water. Just as we use soaps to get grease, which is fat, out of our system, let's say off our hands or out of a piece of cloth, in the body we use fat-soluble products or chemicals that have at one end something that dissolves fat and at the other something that dissolves in water. The water-soluble end can pull the fat into solution. These are transported by combining them with certain proteins that are produced by the liver and we call them "lipoproteins," fat proteins. The transportation in this water-soluble system that we call our body is really done by the lipoproteins.

One of the things they have to carry around is cholesterol, and this is a molecule that we have in huge abundance in our bodies and it is transported to where it is needed. Chemically it is technically an alcohol from a chemist's point of view in the way it is structured. It's not like the alcohol we drink; it's very different. It also has structural similarities to the steroid molecules which are manufactured from cholesterol. Lots of our own hormones are what we call "steroids," which refers to their shape, and we manufacture things like testosterone from cholesterol. We tend to think of cholesterol as something bad that we have to control, but it's a very, very vital structure and molecule in our body.

The lipoproteins in general are arranged into groups by their physical density, which means how quickly they will settle to the bottom of a solution. Unfortunately, it's important we understand the division, so we have to get into a little bit of the nitty gritty about them because you hear about them all the time. You'll get reports from your doctor and we'll talk about raising and lowering them. It's important I think at this point that we understand them.

Low density lipoprotein, or LDL, and very low density, VLDL, are mainly in the body to transport the triglycerides from liver cells to fat cells where they're stored. LDL proteins carry cholesterol in the blood and they deliver it to cells throughout the body for tissue repair, very important for the synthesis of vital chemicals, such as steroid hormones.

But, excessive LDL cholesterol can form around the smooth muscle fibers in our arteries and they form what we're used to calling "fatty plaque," and they increase the risk for coronary artery disease because they narrow our vessels. Hardening of the arteries, or atherosclerosis, is what you may hear it referred to, and this is why we call these two "bad" cholesterol. People with high LDL and VLDL tend to have fatty plaques and this leads to coronary artery disease and heart attacks.

HDL, high density lipoproteins, are in body cells and in the blood stream and they remove excess cholesterol and carry it to the liver for destruction so they can prevent the accumulation of cholesterol in the blood and in the vessels and reduce the risk of coronary artery disease. Therefore we call them the "good" cholesterol. This can actually reverse some of the plaque formation if you have high HDL proteins in there. The best thing that you can do to increase the HDL molecules in your blood is to exercise, not diet. It's a really good option because it has very little to do with what you eat, but much more to do with how much exercise you get.

The total load of the different kinds of cholesterol are really determined, as we mentioned before, by how much we absorb through our diet, via the intestine, which is environment or nurture, and how much is synthesized by our liver cells, genes or nature. I talked to you about the problem I have with that and how I had to solve it. We have dietary and genetic control of cholesterol absorption and its metabolism. Different people have different mechanisms for this. This is reflected in how we can intervene to get the healthiest balance, and here's one place where we have to get a little artificial. Once we've got the right exercise program and once we've got the right diet, we still are going to have a number of patients, just like me, who are still going to have unhealthy levels of LDL and VLDL, and may not have enough HDL.

We can use some drugs that promote the excretion of lipoproteins, the bad ones, into the gut and then out in the feces. We can also prevent the absorption from the intestine through chemicals called "plant stanol esters," just a molecular organic piece that comes from plants, and they can accomplish the same thing preventing it from being absorbed. They've been incorporated for example into some margarine-like products called Benecol and other ones that are coming to market all the time.

Another group of drugs which we've mentioned in the past are called "statins." They block the production of cholesterol in the liver cells and they also may be linked to reducing the inflammation around those plaques. Today actually there's some good information that's telling us that even though the plaques themselves narrow your coronary arteries and other arteries, that it may be equally or even more important that they not have inflammation.

Those fatty plaques are actually seen as an irritant. They set up inflammation, which causes more swelling and narrowing, and just getting rid of the inflammation alone can make improvement.

Every study we get that comes out of this literature, now over millions and millions of patients, many decades of use, now tells us with every single advancing day that this is a great drug when used appropriately and will save lives. I'm very happy to hear that personally from a selfish point of view. The total cholesterol in your body, which is what you get in reports often, is the sum of all the components, the HDL, the LDL, and the VLDL. So low total cholesterol, low LDL, low VLDL coupled, with an elevation of the HDL definitely decreases the risk of coronary artery disease. This is what we want, and I'm going to talk more about the specificity of fat storage a little later and the implications for health.

From this discussion it might seem as if most of the fats were bad except the HDL. That's not the case. They have very, very important functions when we take them in the right amounts and the right kinds of fats. The fats are used as I mentioned for structural molecules, which are part of plasma membranes of every cell. They're used as transport chemicals through the bloodstream, and they're very important in clotting molecules, in nerve insulation. We coat the myelin sheaths of the nerves so that we don't get short circuits. I mentioned that in an earlier lecture.

The triglycerides themselves can be stored inside fat cells. Fat cells can get bigger or smaller depending on the storage. They constitute about 98 percent of the entire body's energy reserves, especially for emergencies. The fats can be stored much more readily than glycogen. We have much less capacity for storing glycogen, which is where we get that glucose rush from. Fat cells under the skin, for example, actually contain about 50 percent of the stored triglycerides. When we run out of glucose, or glycogen, we can switch to burning fat for fuel. It's not as good a fuel, it's not as clean burning a fuel, but it's a good fuel that we can use when we need it.

Fats in our diet now are an important subject. This is going to be as opposed to the fats that are already in our body. We classify our fats that we can eat as saturated or unsaturated. The "saturated fats" is a chemical designation that refers to the fact that when you have a chain of carbon atoms all of them are occupied by hydrogen. In other words, those hydrogen atoms that can appear on different places in the carbon are all full. Those are mainly from animal fats in the diet. That's where we get them.

Saturated and trans-fats, which is the worst of all for your health, are generally solid at room temperature like butter, Crisco, lard. Unsaturated fats have a few of the carbon atoms saturated. There are some spaces in the carbon where a bond is free or left over to be used for something else. They tend to be liquid at room temperatures, and we'll see later how we can make use of this, for example oils from fish that live in very cold water. Solid fats would kill the fish because these fish are coldblooded. Their body temperature drops and if at cold temperatures their fat got solid, they would be frozen and die. They need oils that they can stay mobile while their oil stays liquid, and we can eat those and get the benefits. We'll talk about those later.

There are varieties of unsaturated fats that you've heard a lot about I'm sure. There are monounsaturated fats, which means that just one bond in the whole chain of carbons is missing its hydrogen. There are polyunsaturated fats, which means some number more than one bond is unfilled with hydrogen.

Unsaturated fats, particularly monounsaturated fats, the kind we find in avocado, are very, very healthy, probably the healthiest of them all. Many healthy, unsaturated fats are typically as I said liquids, and the ones that come to mind are flaxseed oil, canola oil, and olive oil especially, very, very healthy fat for you. Trans-fats, which I mentioned just briefly earlier, is a designation that really refers to a chemical arrangement of that fatty molecule. They all increase the risk for coronary heart disease. They increase the levels of the bad LDL cholesterol, and they lower the level of the good HDL cholesterol.

The best course for you is to not even think about them. Get them out of your diet completely. Almost every scientific agency that has studied this, points out that trans-fats of either animal or plant origin are not essential to human health in any way. Also beware of the term that you'll see on labels "partially hydrogenated vegetable oils." That's where they take an unsaturated fat and they chemically force hydrogen back onto them. They are unhealthy.

There's really no place for the trans-fatty acids in our diet. They do not help you and they cause harm. You might ask, "Why are they in our foods?" Partial hydrogenation, it's what you see on the label, extends the shelf life of the product and it reduces the need for refrigeration. It's also less expensive than semi-solid oils that are used in baking. But the widespread scientific and political consumer outcries about this have made great headway in trying to get them out of our foods. There are some countries in Europe now where they are completely illegal in foods.

I want to talk very quickly about proteins in our diet. They're generally used as enzymes as one function, as transportation of oxygen such as hemoglobin, antibodies, clotting molecules, in muscle fibers, in structural components like hair, nails, bones. They're basically made of a chain of amino acids, which are linked together and we can make some of these amino acids in our body. The important information here is that we have something called "essential amino acids." Those are the ones we cannot make, we have to eat them.

Of the 20 amino acids we need to make human proteins, ten of them are essential. Plants happily can synthesize them so we can get all we need by eating plants or other animals that have them by eating plants too. Nutritionists also talk about complete protein source. This means it has all the essential amino acids and there are incomplete ones that may lack some of the essential amino acids.

What we can do is combine the two incomplete sources such as rice and beans and make a complete source. I'll talk to you a lot about that in the future. In emergencies, your body is terrific. It can just take glucose, some other amino acids, mix them all up and come out with exactly what we want, and we can take the amino acids and reverse those and bring them back as glucose for energy, called "gluconeogenesis," new glucose birth is what it means literally.

During digestion proteins are broken down into their forms and then they're absorbed and oxidized and they can burn as energy to make that ATP/ADP cycle work, or they can make new proteins, or they can be converted. Note again that all these molecules are absolutely interconvertible, the body has a terrific way through evolution of getting emergency sources of exactly what it needs.

I'm going to talk to you for a few minutes about the food pyramids and then we'll move into the molecular specifics of nutrition. There's a new food pyramid from the USDA that's come out in recent years. They call it "MyPyramid." You can find it at their website. Basically the pyramids encourage foods that are geared to specific caloric needs. They have added a new category now called "exercise." The food pyramids are generally arranged so you have bars going vertically up the pyramid, and different colors specify the kinds of foods they're including. Each group should be eaten daily and the wider the band on the pyramid the more of that product you should be eating. The widths are just a guide to the portion size, not an exact recommendation. They're now using cups and ounces instead of servings. If we compare

Latin American, Asian, and Mediterranean food pyramids, which you can find in the *Old Ways* book in our bibliography, we see they're basically the same in proportions. We have differences in which grains and vegetables are eaten in those countries, but in the proportion of grains, fruits, and meats they tend to be the same. They would still occupy the same proportion if we moved to another country and there's also a vegetarian pyramid for people who don't eat any meat or fish at all.

What's a healthy diet? Basically they've got to include a little bit of everything, the lowest amount of saturated fats, lots of fruits and veggies, lots of whole grains, and then some variation in all the different food categories. It's generally low in sugars, in cholesterol, in salt, and very low in saturated fat. The food pyramids are not designed to address specific diseases. In general it's just a sensible guideline that avoids going to extremes.

The next time we come back we're going to remind ourselves again about some of our guidelines like moderation, moderation, moderation; about the Goldilocks rule; and about the one-degree change. We'll continue our exploring some of the optimal food groups and how they can provide us lifelong health.

The Role of Vitamins
Lecture 13

A safe rule of thumb for me—if you want to look for some guidance— would be not to go over twice the daily RDA in your vitamin supplement in most cases. I'm speaking of supplements here, not the food. ... You're generally safer getting almost all your exposure to vitamins in whole foods.

Vitamins are nutrients our bodies require from an external source because we cannot manufacture them ourselves. Vitamins are a group of 13 organic chemical compounds that are required for normal growth and development. Their functions include acting as hormone messengers (vitamin D), regulators of tissue growth and cell differentiation (vitamin A), and **antioxidants** (vitamins A, C, and E). A vitamer is one of two or more related chemical substances that fulfills the same specific vitamin function. Vitamin supplements are any or all of the 13 defined vitamins taken as a pill or injection. Supplements in general are taken to improve nutrition in areas where we are deficient.

Among the 13 vitamins, 4 are soluble in fat: A, D, E, and K. Those in the vitamin B complex and vitamin C are water soluble. Water-soluble vitamins are easily excreted, which means that regular intake is important. The fat-soluble vitamins require fats to transport them through the gastrointestinal wall so they can get into the bloodstream. The recommended daily allowances (RDA) refer to the average need for a healthy adult.

As far as we know, there is no scientific difference between natural and synthetic vitamins. But there is a difference in the fact that when you get most of your vitamins from foods, there may be other chemicals acting in synergy with the single vitamin.

The Women's Health Initiative Study followed 160,000 postmenopausal women over the course of eight years. Forty percent of the women in the study used multivitamins, but no association was found between multivitamin use and reduction in the risks of various cancers or the overall death rate.

Additional studies have shown that even moderately high doses of vitamin supplements can cause serious consequences. For example, high doses of vitamin E actually increased the risk of dying in patients with heart disease. High doses of vitamin C have been shown to offer no benefit for preventing common colds. In fact, a study published in the *Archives of Internal Medicine* found that there were no benefits confirmed for multivitamin consumption in 10 categories, including the prevention of blood clots, reduction in the risk of breast or colon cancer, and so on.

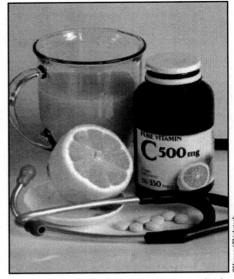

Vitamin C in high doses does not assist in preventing common colds.

With a few exceptions, the vitamins and nutrients from whole foods are generally sufficient to prevent vitamin deficiencies. The exceptions include B$_{12}$ injections sometimes given to elderly patients, folic acid given to pregnant women, and vitamin D plus calcium given to postmenopausal women.

If you feel you must take a vitamin supplement beyond what you're eating in a whole-food diet, then limit yourself to maintenance doses. Take a good-quality multivitamin and, perhaps, a mineral supplement without exceeding the RDA. Be aware, too, that infants and children need specialized vitamin care. Patients who are taking medication for heart disease or kidney disease, are on anticoagulants, or are on steroids should note that supplements can interact dangerously with many medications. Cancer patients should talk to their doctors about taking supplements. Finally, when you choose a supplement, look for some certification, such as the National Science Foundation International label or the Consumer Labs seal of approval. ■

antioxidants: Substances that may protect cells by neutralizing the free radicals that damage cells and tissue.

vitamins: Organic chemical compounds required by the body from external sources because they cannot be manufactured internally.

1. How is a supplement different from a vitamin? What purposes do supplements and vitamins serve, and can they be over- or underutilized?

2. Discuss the vitamin-related scientific trials covered in the lecture. Which had results that surprised you?

The Role of Vitamins
Lecture 13—Transcript

Welcome back again. Today, we'll move onto one of the micronutrients that we mentioned earlier. Remember that we're going to be talking about whole foods. But, to understand nutrition, it's necessary to break the components down into pieces that we can understand so we can see how they function. In this lecture, we'll focus on vitamins, which are nutrients our bodies absolutely require from an external source because we cannot manufacture them ourselves. There are nutrients that, in small amounts, are critical for health and well-being. Vitamins are one of them. In the next lecture, we'll focus on supplements.

There is some confusion when we talk about a number of terms. We talk about vitamins and vitamin supplements. We talk about supplements and dietary supplements as well as the meanings of "organic" or "natural." Let's just stop here for a minute and define them as best we can so we can talk about them without confusion. I mentioned before that there were two meanings of "organic." The one I touched on in the last lecture was the chemical definition. The "organic" that we refer to in the biology of compounds or molecules that are found in nature and which have a carbon base is primarily the one used by the chemists. These may be natural or they may be synthetic. Some of them overlap and confuse the definition. In nutrition and farming, we talk about plants and animal products which are defined by the method of farming—including many rules, such as no use of chemical pesticides and no use of chemical fertilizer. We're going to talk a lot about this. This is one of my favorite subjects.

Getting back to vitamins, basically, these are a group of 13 organic chemical compounds. They're defined by nutritional scientists as being required for normal growth and development. They're necessary in the diet because we can't make them in any sufficient quantity at all. We also classify them as to their function in the body rather than their chemistry or their origin in nature. The functions include: acting as hormone messengers, such as vitamin D; regulators of tissue growth and cell differentiation, as in vitamin A; and then antioxidants, such as vitamin A, C, and E. There is overlap in what they do.

There is a whole range of enzymes which regulate chemical reactions, too. These are the vitamin B complex that we refer to as one group.

There's another definition you probably want to know and that's called a "vitamer." It's one of two or more related chemical substances that fulfill the same specific vitamin function. It's a matter, again, of biologic activity, not molecular structure. Vitamers can also be inter-converted in the body, one into another, so the body can get what it needs at a particular time. For example, "vitamin A" is a generic description of several vitamins which carry out certain functions. But, they may include chemicals such as retinal, retinol, and some of keratinoids—which are, by definition, vitamers of vitamin A.

Where it gets a little fuzzy is when we say "vitamin supplements." These are any or all of the 13 defined vitamins when you take them as an extra dose, or a pill, or an injection—as we sometimes give the B vitamins—aside from the ones we get in our diets. It's a complicated process and a complicated subject. It gets even more confusing when we talk of the supplements and dietary supplements. Supplements are what we take to improve nutrition in areas where we are either deficient in that the foods we eat don't contain enough of the substance naturally—such as iodine if the local salt doesn't have enough iodine in it—or if there is a deficiency in that we just don't eat enough of the right foods. For example, a lack of omega-3 fatty acids in diets where there are not enough fish sources or other sources for the omega 3s. I will talk a lot about omega 3s later. It is also when it is taken in excess of the diet with the aim to improving some deficient function in the body. For example, someone who doesn't make enough thyroid hormone might take a thyroid hormone supplement. Again, it can be taken in excess of the diet to improve beyond normal function such as muscle-building protein supplements. We'll talk about more of that later and I bet you can already guess what I'm going to say about it.

Some supplements, such as calcium, are needed to maintain, for example, the declining function that occurs with age such as bone loss. They cannot be considered vitamins by definition because this is a simple element— calcium is not an organic compound, it doesn't contain any carbon. That is it for the supplements at this point. I'll talk much more about it later, in the next lecture.

Because vitamins are species specific—some animals can make their own vitamin C for example, while we cannot—we will confine the discussion only to human vitamin requirements. We're not going to talk about animals at all. There's a classification that actually is fairly important. That is whether vitamins are water soluble or fat soluble. In humans, as I said, there are 13 vitamins and 4 of them are soluble in fat. Those are A, D, E, and K. If you remember those, you can just remember that all the rest are soluble in water. Those include vitamin B complex, which are eight in number, and vitamin C. Those are the water soluble ones. Again, A, D, E, and K are for fat.

The consequences of this difference in fat or water solubility—which means dissolvability—is that water-soluble vitamins have several characteristics. They are very easily excreted, as many of you may have noticed when you urinate about an hour after taking vitamins. You'll see that your urine takes on a much more intense yellow color because you are excreting a lot of colorful vitamins which you paid a lot of money for. They're not easily stored in the body so a regular intake is important. We can't go too long without taking them in. It doesn't mean that they can't reach toxic levels. But, we have much better mechanisms to prevent that than we do with fat-soluble vitamins. We'll get to that as we move along through the topic.

The fat-soluble vitamins—again, A, D, E, and K—require fats to transport them through the gastrointestinal wall so they can get into the bloodstream. Remember, like things dissolve in like things; fats dissolve in fats. It's better, for example, if they're taken with a slightly fatty meal or they have other fat elements in the vitamin. Since they're stored in fat as well, they can accumulate in the body. They are more likely to lead to possible hypervitaminosis diseases in high doses. "Hypervitaminosis" means too much vitamin, and there are diseases of hypervitaminosis. Therefore, they're more likely to reach toxic levels if you megadose. Remember my friends with the orange hands from eating too much keratein—that's a case of megadosing, a case of hypervitaminosis as well, fortunately one that is not very toxic.

You probably are all familiar with the designation of "RDA" that's on vitamin bottles. This means recommended daily allowances. This comes from research done over a wide variety of populations. It refers, really, only to the average need for a healthy adult. There's a very different RDA for children. That's important; you don't want your children taking your vitamins. The RDA may not be enough if you have special needs—in other words, if you have some illness that's using up vitamins, are under increased stress, or increased requirements, for example, from high level athletic activity. Going slightly over the RDA is probably not a problem as the body can deal with the excess by either inactivating it or excreting it most of the time. There's a lot of leeway. But again, I want to emphasize that I think megadoses are an entirely different matter. There are toxic effects of extreme overdoses of vitamins. Almost any substance that you take into your body can be toxic at some point, even water. If you chugalug enormous amounts of water in a short period of time, it can actually be fatal. It's been proven, unfortunately, too many times.

A safe rule of thumb for me, if you want to look for some guidance, would be not to go over twice the daily RDA in your vitamin supplement in most cases. I'm speaking of supplements here, not the food. It's a lot harder to overdose when you're taking vitamins in your food. It's possible—again, my friends with their orange hands—but it's a little harder. You're generally safer getting almost all your exposure to vitamins in whole foods. If you have special concerns about your health, then you really need to talk to your doctor and make an individual decision.

We're going to look at a few of the critical issues for some of the vitamins. I've included the resources for you in the bibliography and some of the websites as well as a general chart in the guidebook. I want to talk for a minute about the argument about synthetic vitamins versus natural vitamins and the controversy it has engendered in some of the health-food journals and articles. As far as we know, there is absolutely no scientific difference between natural and synthetic vitamins. They have exactly the same chemical structure in supplemental form as they do in foods in natural form. The molecules are exactly the same. There is a difference in the fact that when you get most of your vitamins from foods, there may be other chemicals acting in synergy with the single vitamin. Synergy, as you may recall, is

179

when the total is more than the sum of the two parts. It's two and two is five. But, this is true of many, many chemicals in our body. We talked about the creatines which I will probably get to again. There are over 60 of them. It's a very important point to remember. The synergy of the whole food is going to provide something for you that a single supplement can't. It's going to give you something extra.

I spoke about the synergistic relationship in an earlier lecture with regard to whole foods, but claims that food-derived vitamins are somehow safer or better than synthetic vitamins are just not backed by science. When you go into a store, there's usually just shelves full of different companies trying to sell you vitamins. Often you see the majority of them may have some from whole-food sources and then broken down and condensed into a pill. They usually require that you take many more pills per day to get the same dose, but there's nothing anywhere in the science that tells us that these are actually better for you.

We get back to Hamlet's great question—to take vitamins or not to take vitamins; that is the question. As it is now, about 50 percent or more of Americans take vitamins and/or supplements on a daily basis. For this, they spend about $20 billion a year. There have been lots of studies. The problem is it's very difficult to find good, double-blind, randomized, controlled studies that show any unequivocal benefit for vitamin supplementation. The data from dietary journals that people keep when they're on these studies— or from their memory—are very, very inaccurate. They are notoriously inaccurate. If you try to think back on what you ate on Monday, when it's Friday, it'd be very hard to replicate that. We know the information is very, very soft. Vitamin supplement studies also are very skewed by differences in what others food sources are being eaten. The patient takes a vitamin and has another general diet. We don't know where those other foods are providing some of the gaps or filling in on vitamins they have been missing in the study.

I want to introduce you to the Women's Health Initiative Study, an enormous study we're going to run into again and again in the course. This is a small branch of it which was devoted to vitamins. In this study, there were 160,000 post-menopausal women. They were studied for eight years. That's an enormous study—very well controlled, very tightly structured. Forty percent of the women used multivitamins. What they found out, in analyzing it later, was that there was no association between multivitamin use and reducing the risks of a whole number of diseases. These included breast cancer, lung cancer, colorectal cancer, endometrial cancer, which is the lining of the uterus, ovarian cancers, cardiovascular heart disease, or even just the overall death rate. It did appear to show that women eating a nutrient-rich diet, with lots of fruits and vegetables, did have lower rates of heart disease and cancer than those who were on multivitamins with a more conventional diet. Additional studies outside this one show that possible serious harm from vitamin supplements can occur in even moderately high doses.

The following that I'm going to tell you about and list for you all came from peer-reviewed journals. This includes mostly high doses. Vitamin C and E for heart disease had absolutely no meaningful benefit. The John Hopkins School of Medicine reviewed 19 trials, 135,000 patients—very big study. High doses here of vitamin E, which was greater than 400 international units a day, increased the risk of dying during the four-year study period. Not only did it not protect them, it increased the risk of dying. Fifteen-thousand male doctors took vitamin E and C for 10 years with no effect at all on cancer rates.

High doses of vitamin E plus other vitamins and minerals yielded, in some studies, a 6 percent increased death rate. Vitamin E increased the risk for heart failure by approximately 13 percent. That's an enormous increase. Vitamin E again, and selenium for prostate cancer prevention; Vitamin E we already know is a vitamin, selenium is a trace element found in tiny, tiny amounts in foods and in soil and we only need tiny amounts. It was thought to be protective for prostate cancer, as was vitamin E. It was put into a double-blind, crossover, peer-reviewed study. It was found that, in this case, they actually had to terminate the study prematurely because very early on, there were concerns that the treatment risks far outweighed the benefit. Patients were either actually getting more illness or they were dying sooner.

The big one was among smokers and asbestos workers. These are because both those groups have a high incidence of lung cancer. They gave them high doses of beta-carotene and vitamin A. We talked before about beta-carotene—this great antioxidant, which it is, in foods—then our comments about how the other carotenes may be very important. The beta-carotene alone might not give you the benefit. What else might it give you? We didn't know. This study showed that, after the period of time in the study, which was several years, 28 percent had increased risk for lung cancer. It didn't protect them at all. Their risk actually went up. Twenty-six percent had an increased risk of heart disease related death. They died of heart attacks or arrhythmia, rhythm disturbances. This was also terminated prematurely because of the results. They found they were doing something dangerous.

Then, we get into the whole issue of vitamin C trials for treating common colds. Common colds are a viral illness, so the idea was somehow that vitamin C could increase your resistance. This is what the terminology has long been. We are going to increase your resistance and stop the virus from affecting you. Remember that colds are caught by getting viruses from other people. It has nothing to do with the cold, because it has nothing to do with temperature. The reason we get more colds—which is why we named them this—during the winter is that we tend to be shut indoors more. Fewer windows are open and there's less ventilation. Patients or rooms get higher concentrations of the viruses, but it really is not anything to do with the cold.

There were two dozen studies that were reviewed. In none of these studies was there a benefit for preventing the incidence of common colds. It's interesting that they also, in some studies, took patients and sat them outside in wet bathing suits in cold weather—just what our mother told us never to do. There was no incidence in whether they got colds or not. What they really could do to give people colds was to put common cold virus in the noses of some people and have them sit down together for an evening of cards. In the end, everybody got infected from the viruses because of transmission.

In this, there was another interesting finding which I think is absolutely fascinating. There was a 50 percent reduction in colds among extreme athletes and soldiers that were serving in very, very cold conditions. We're now talking about well below zero, not just a cold day, and under enormous physical stress. There's something that the protection from vitamin C gave these people. We don't know what it was, we don't know how it worked, but that's undergoing further studies.

From the *New England Journal of Medicine*—really one of the great peer-reviewed journals in the world and one I read before I read anything else—vitamins don't benefit patients with established vascular disease. It was thought that we could help people whose vessels were under stress and weren't doing well. It doesn't seem to be the case. The *Archives of Internal Medicine,* another very good journal, found that there were no benefits confirmed for multivitamin consumption in 10 categories. Those included among the 10 were in preventing fatal or dangerous blood clots, in reducing the risk of breast or colon cancer, in reducing the risk of heart attack or overall mortality, and reducing the risk of stroke. The vitamins and the nutrients from whole foods are generally sufficient to prevent vitamin deficiencies. We saw that in the Women's Health initiative, as well as in the studies in the Mediterranean diet—which we'll talk about later and which I think you'll find very, very interesting.

A few exceptions to this rule might be needed, and I want to mention them. Vitamin B_{12}, often given by injection, is sometimes needed in elderly patients who tend to lose the absorption capability. The vitamin B, especially B_{12}, is absorbed in the last few inches of your small intestine before the food goes into the colon. For some reason, probably an aging vascular system, these patients don't have the ability to absorb it as well. This is also the reason we tend to give it by injection in elderly people because giving it by mouth might not help as much.

Folic acid is another one of the B-complex vitamins which is very essential for women of child-bearing age, especially if they are preparing to get pregnant or preparing to give birth. This is another exception to the rule. Vitamin D and calcium is another big exception. I'll talk more about it in future lectures. Women—especially post-menopausal women—are at risk for osteoporosis, softening of the bones, and therefore fractures. They will benefit from supplemental vitamin D plus calcium. I'll get into this a lot later. It is probably good for older men as well.

In conclusion, I think we want to look back at all the details of these studies and say that, in a perfect world, we could and we probably should get all our vitamin requirements in our diet alone. We should not need any expensive supplements or numbers of pills through the day to get protection. Vitamin deficiencies in this country are so rare that I can honestly tell you—in 30 years, I never saw a single case of vitamin deficiency disease. Even though people may have slightly worse or slightly better health because of some vitamin, we never see things like beriberi, pellagra, or scurvy. These were diseases that were recognized long ago. Captain Cook and Captain Bligh knew to make their sailors eat onions and limes all the time onboard ship to prevent scurvy, which is a shortage of vitamin C. Yet, they didn't even know what a vitamin was. However, in our world, not everyone can or will get all their nutrients from their food. It just isn't going to happen and it's not realistic.

What I would recommend is that for you—and this is just a suggestion— if you really feel you must take a vitamin supplement beyond what you're eating in this whole-food diet that I hope you'll adopt, then limit yourself to maintenance doses. This is a program where you have a good quality multivitamin and perhaps a mineral supplement along with it, without exceeding the daily recommended allowances. Then, you would have a baseline level. You'd have a safety net. You'd be unlikely to exceed the toxic doses at the top, but you'd have a baseline at the bottom to cushion you if your diet should fail to give you what you need. However, these vitamins should be balanced with a whole food diet. They shouldn't be taken to make up for the gaps. They're not to be used instead of food or healthy lifestyle. Pregnant or breastfeeding women should actually be on special vitamins. That should be a decision between you and your doctor. Sometimes a prenatal vitamin support would be specifically prescribed for them by their local doctor. Women trying to become pregnant should take special care to avoid high doses. There have been a number of cases of problems in women taking megadoses while they are pregnant or while they are trying to become pregnant.

Infants and children need absolutely specialized vitamin care. You should follow the recommendations of your pediatricians to the letter. Patients taking special medication for heart disease or kidney disease, who may be on anticoagulants, including Aspirin, or on steroids, should always be aware that supplements can interact very dangerously with many medications. You need to look into this. The more medicines you're taking, the more careful you'll have to be. In patients undergoing surgery in the near future, supplements can cause bleeding. I'll go into those a little bit later, but again, this just means you should be alert.

Cancer patients—supplements could increase the growth rate of cancer cells. This is kind of counterintuitive, but cancer cells like supplements too, just as normal cells like supplements. Talk to your doctor if you have cancer.

Alcoholism's another problem. Alcoholics have very specific needs for vitamin supplements because their nutrition is usually markedly deficient and they require extra support. They generally have bad diets. They have inadequate intake of nutrients. There is also a problem with absorption in the intestine. They have liver injuries because alcohol is an absolute toxin for the liver so they have to be very closely in touch with their doctors.

When, finally, you decide you're going to have a supplement that you need, then look for some certification. There's too many out there that may not have the proper ingredients. Look for something like the National Science Foundation International label, US Pharmacopeia label, or Consumer Labs seal of approval. These will tell you that the vitamins or the supplements that you're taking do contain the ingredients that the label says are there. The product also would probably not contain any contaminants or potentially harmful ingredients. What they don't certify is that the substances are good for you or that they're in the right dose for you. I tend to buy only products produced in the United States. It's not about politics, it's not about economics. Products from abroad are not necessarily regulated for toxic ingredients. Products, recently, from China have been a big issue in this regard. For me, avoid megadoses of any vitamin or any supplement. Try, if you can, to think about getting all your nutrition from whole foods.

This concludes the section on the first of our key micronutrients, vitamins. Next time, we'll look forward and focus on supplements.

The Role of Supplements
Lecture 14

> All the evidence points to the direction of relying on our food; capsules and supplements—absolutely do not rely on them. ... Pig out on carrots, sweet potatoes, chard if you like it, asparagus, papaya, prunes, oranges—the whole vast array of foods that are delicious and are good for you.

In the last lecture, we talked about the differences between vitamins and supplements. In this lecture, we'll focus on nutrients and chemicals that when added to the diet might lower the risk for some health problems and might improve overall bodily function.

Dietary supplements do not need to be approved by the FDA, but it is illegal to advertise supplements as a treatment or cure for any specific disease or condition. Manufacturers can, however, make claims that the supplement aids or supports some particular function.

Antioxidants are one major category of supplements. As we've seen, **oxidation** reactions can create free radicals, which are part of normal host defenses but can also cause cell damage. Most of the time, our bodies can handle the free radical load, but excessive production can damage cells and cause **oxidative stress** (the elevation of free radicals beyond the body's capability to neutralize them). Antioxidants halt these chain reactions by neutralizing free radicals and their intermediates.

We have both internal and external naturally occurring antioxidants. Glutathione is one, along with vitamins C and E and numerous enzymes. Fruits and vegetables, whole grains, and nuts are dietary sources of antioxidants. The sources of destructive free radicals include ultraviolet and other forms of radiation, toxins, and pollutants. Free radicals contribute to the development of many diseases, but recent research suggests that megadoses of antioxidants taken as supplements cannot prevent heart disease or diabetes. Additionally, large doses may be harmful.

Oxidative stress plays a clear role in cardiovascular disease, but controlled studies with antioxidant supplements show no reduction in the risk of developing heart disease or in the rate of progression of the disease. If a diet rich in antioxidants is beneficial but supplements are not, what's going on? The theory is that other molecules in fruits and vegetables improve cardiovascular health in patients with diets high in these foods.

Calcium is the most abundant mineral in the body and is involved in muscle contraction and nerve conduction, among other processes and functions. Of course, calcium is used to prevent osteoporosis, but it has also been suggested that it may have value for cardiovascular health and cancer prevention. Conclusive evidence in this regard is not yet available. Vitamin D and magnesium may be prescribed with calcium. Calcium sources in food include dairy products, dark-green leafy vegetables, and nuts and seeds.

> **The message is, get as many of your antioxidants from whole foods, highly colored fruits and veggies especially, and don't megadose on the supplements.**

Fiber is basically the indigestible part of plant food that creates bulk in the digestive system. It keeps the bowels soft and may help eliminate toxic wastes. Some soft evidence suggests that fiber may offer some protection from heart disease, reduce the risk of colon and breast cancer, and reduce blood sugar in diabetics. I recommend drinking about a tablespoon of powered psyllium in berry juice daily as a fiber supplement.

Herbal supplements are those derived from plants. Common ones include ginkgo biloba, ginseng, and echinacea. Very little science backs up the claims of these supplements. Again, many legally sold dietary supplements are not required to obtain FDA approval for safety or effectiveness. Furthermore, many supplements have serious lethal potential when taken in large doses or with prescribed drugs. ■

fiber: The indigestible part of plant food (roughage) that creates bulk in the digestive system. It absorbs water and promotes defecation; may aid in eliminating toxic wastes.

herbal supplements: Supplements derived from plants.

oxidation: A process whereby electrons are transferred from one molecule or atom to another, creating free radicals. Free radicals and oxidation reactions are a necessary part of normal host defenses, but excess oxidation reactions are damaging.

oxidative stress: The elevation of free radicals beyond the body's capability to neutralize them to safe levels. Excessive oxidative stress damages the cells and tissues, specifically the mitochondria.

Questions to Consider

1. Do you take supplements or vitamins? If so, why? If not, why not?

2. What are antioxidants, and why do they matter to your health? What are some natural food sources that are high in antioxidants?

The Role of Supplements
Lecture 14—Transcript

Welcome back. Today, we'll examine the other major group of nutrients—supplements, and their role in a healthy diet. We'll look at the various foods where we can obtain these nutrients without actually going to supplemental pills. Again, we want to remind ourselves what actually is a dietary supplement. In the last lecture, we talked about the differences between vitamins and supplements and some of the confusion over the terms. Here, we're going to focus on the nutrients and chemicals that when added to the diet might lower your risk of some health problems—like osteoporosis, arthritis, cardiovascular disease, and so on—and might improve the vital function of the body overall. This will explicitly eliminate vitamins from the discussions. Everything else will be fair game.

First, physicians' prescriptions are generally not needed if you want to buy a supplement, or even a vitamin. The FDA usually categorizes supplements as a food. Therefore, they cannot be scrutinized necessarily as much as other categories of drugs. This can be good and bad because it makes them more accessible, but it keeps them out of the eyes of the regulators of quality and safety. Dietary supplements, like food, do not need to be approved by the FDA. It is illegal to advertise a dietary supplement as treatment or cure for any specific disease or condition. But, the manufacturers can make claims regarding structure and/or function. They can say that the supplement aids or supports some particular body function. For example, "glucosamine helps maintain healthy joints"—even if there's no proof that it does any such thing. What they can't do is claim that it is a cure for a specific disease. So in this case they couldn't say it cures osteoarthritis which might be giving you the pain in your joints.

There are major categories of supplements and I'll try to touch on the most important ones as far as we're concerned. The first are the antioxidants. We've already talked about oxidation reactions that create free radicals which can cause cell damage. Remember from the earlier lectures, that in a process called "oxidation," electronics are transferred from one molecule or atom to another. Recall that the free radicals and oxidation reactions are a necessary part of normal host defenses like apoptosis—cell suicide—destruction of foreign chemicals, and organisms such as germs or viruses. But, excess oxidation reactions are damaging. These are increased in metabolic activity that's very high and more free radicals are generated. Exercise and fever, for example, both release excess free radicals. Exercise does it as a normal part of energy metabolism and its production and consumption, while fever is abnormal. It may produce more free radicals over a longer period of time as long as the fever persists.

Most of the time, our bodies can handle the free radical load. It's the excessive production and the failure to deal with these excess free radicals that damage cells, and what we now call—and I want you to remember—as "oxidative stress." We're going to come back to it a lot. Antioxidants halt these chain reactions by neutralizing the free radicals and their intermediates. There are a huge amount of bioavailable antioxidants in naturally occurring food. That's where I want to see us get them from. I'm going to talk about them later. For now, I want to confine most of this discussion to the antioxidants supplied as supplements, mostly as pills or as liquids.

Common antioxidant molecules in nature are often what are called "polyphenols." These, again, are a complex organic molecule. They're called "polyphenols" because they have a number of phenol rings attached, which is just a chemical designation. They're very complicated molecules. We have both internal and external naturally occurring antioxidants. Glutathione is one, vitamin C is another, vitamin E, and lots and lots of enzymes. Fruits and vegetables, whole gains, and nuts contain dietary sources of the antioxidants which we can use as well. vitamin C and E we've mentioned, selenium, and zinc is another one we haven't come across yet that is another element as opposed to an organic molecule.

Remember that these chemicals evolve in the plants to protect them from stress and from environmental attack. We just benefit by eating them. A whole group is designated as "phytonutrients." This means that they come from plants. These are called "flavonoids," "carotinoids," and "beta-carotene," and all those other carotenoids I pointed to earlier. The destructive exogenous free radicals—which are the ones that come from outside—include ultraviolet radiation, other forms of radiation, toxins, and pollutants. The free radicals contribute to the development of a lot of our diseases including the whole inflammatory group of disease such as arthritis, of atherosclerosis—hardening of the arteries—and its inflammation, cancer, diabetes, and so on.

Research recently suggests that the megadoses of the exogenous antioxidants taken as supplements cannot prevent diseases such as heart disease or diabetes. Additionally, extra large doses might even be harmful. People who eat diets rich in fruits and vegetables high in antioxidants definitely have lower rates of heart disease and neurologic diseases such a brain disease. But, then, there's this leap of logic. People think that if a little is good, then more might be better. We now know that adding more antioxidants in the form of supplements to prevent or cure the conditions is definitely not established. It may not necessarily be better. It's certainly found to be worse in some cases. It's not nice to fool Mother Nature. We have to come back to that again.

Recall the study showing that the increase in lung cancer deaths that occurred after the trials of several of the antioxidants, especially beta-carotene. Let's look at a few really interesting facts. In cardiovascular disease, especially, the clear role of oxidative stress has been proven over and over again. But, controlled studies with supplements show absolutely no reduction in the risk of developing heart disease or slowing the progression in someone who already has heart disease. If a diet rich in antioxidants does help and the supplements do not, what's the possible mechanism that's going on here? The theory is the one we've brought up before—that the other molecules in the fruits and vegetables such as the flavonoids or the polyphenols, or a complex mixture of the molecules, improve the cardiovascular health in those patients with diets high in fruits and vegetables. They may be working as a team. We're back to synergy. Remember, there are probably more than 600 carotenes in the world, just to name one group. At least 60 of them are important to human health. By singling out beta-carotene, we're probably missing the synergistic benefit and we're getting some bad effects as we saw.

In an exercise study, they found a very interesting anomaly. Exercise, as we know, generates a lot of the free radicals. The body responds to the free radical damage by up regulating the molecules that it already has to deal with oxidative stress. But, extra antioxidants given as vitamin C or E appear just to bypass whatever it is that generates our normal body response. We're going entirely around what we would like to use by giving these extra vitamin supplements.

The message is—get as many of your antioxidants from whole foods, highly colored fruits and veggies especially, and don't megadose on the supplements. For example, many of them that are out there are represented by things like lycopene which we haven't mentioned yet. It's a carotenoid which we can find in very high concentrations in the blood of healthy people. It's also high in tomatoes. It is associated with protection against prostate cancer. Lutein, which is another carotenoid, is associated with protection against what is called "age-associated macular degeneration." This is a disease that causes blindness in a lot of older people. Strive for the widest range of colored fruits and vegetables that you can get. Don't forget the non-colored fruits and vegetables, too. They have a lot of chemicals in them that can be very helpful to you.

All the evidence points to the direction of relying on our food; capsules and supplements—absolutely do not rely on them. Not that they're terribly bad for you, but generally, they're not going to do it. Stick with the whole foods. Pig out on carrots, sweet potatoes, chard if you like it, asparagus, papaya, prunes, oranges—the whole vast array of foods that are delicious and are good for you. The choices are absolutely endless and it's simple. It's also usually cheaper than the supplements. We'll talk in detail about where, how, and which fruits and vegetables to eat in the next lectures. You can also refer to the website of the Office of Dietary Supplements which is listed in our bibliography. It's an excellent resource.

I'd like to move on to calcium which is the most abundant mineral in our body. Ninety-five percent of our total body calcium is in bones and in our teeth. Less than 1 percent of it is in the blood, muscle, and intercellular fluid—which is the fluid that lines our tissues that is not contained inside the cells. They have very important roles. Calcium is involved in muscle contraction, nerve conduction, blood vessel elasticity and softness, and secretion of hormones and enzymes—hugely important elements. Constant levels are maintained in the body fluids and tissues to very, very finely monitored levels. The way it's done is the calcium is either mobilized from the bones or put back in the bones. Hormones regulate this and measure it very carefully. I'll talk more about that when we get to osteoporosis.

Calcium, in nature, is usually found as a chemical salt combined with either a carbonate—calcium carbonate—or a chloride—like sodium chloride—except in this case, it's calcium chloride, or a citrate. Most of the prescribed supplements for prevention and/or treatment of osteoporosis contain one of these. We'll talk about them later, but there's been much research on its value also in cardiovascular health and cancer prevention. The science there is a little soft. We're just not sure about that one. It's available in lots of forms in nature to you. Choosing the form can be important. For most people, it's not too critical. But, in some cases it is—for example, people who may have low or absent stomach acid. This is because calcium carbonate is much better dissolved in an acid environment. If you're taking antacid medications or are on one of the newer proton-pump inhibitors like Nexium or omeprazole for acid reflux, then you might be better off buying the citrate because that'll be better absorbed than the calcium carbonate form.

Doses are very important. This is especially important in calcium because of a peculiarity. Our bodies really have trouble absorbing more than about 500 to 600 milligrams of calcium at a time. The usual daily dose recommended as a supplement is around 1,000 to 1,200, so these should be taken as separate doses in separate times of the day. My opinion is that you should also separate calcium from other medications. Take them at a different time. Calcium has a propensity, sometimes, to latch on to certain other medications and it may inactivate them. If you're taking vitamins, if you're going to take them, or prescribed medications in the morning, wait an hour or so. Then, take your calcium. Do the same in the evening.

Vitamin D is also usually prescribed along with calcium as a supplement because it helps the action and the absorption of calcium. It's generally the prescription for osteoporosis. We try to aim for a total calcium intake, including food, of about 1,500 milligrams a day—just a little bit more than you would be getting from the supplement. Women who are worried about osteoporosis also take about 800 units of vitamin D, which is a bit more than the usual recommended daily allowance.

Data on protein intake and bone density is a little bit conflicting. Some studies say that high protein intake may lead to lowering the risk of hip fractures, for example, in patients with osteoporosis. Other studies say that high protein intake may increase bone reabsorption of calcium and therefore lead to more fractures. Right now, we're not recommending any changes in normal protein intake.

Magnesium supplements improve bone density versus the placebo group which, over the same period of time, actually lost bone density. But, magnesium deficiency is not really very common all by itself. You usually get enough magnesium.

Calcium is often combined, however, if you're going to take the supplement, with magnesium, and probably—again, probably, because we don't know— the optimal ratio is somewhere about one to one, calcium to magnesium, or two to one, calcium to magnesium, more calcium. Really, weight-bearing exercise—one of the things we do in walking, jogging, and things we do while we're standing up—is an absolute critical adjunct to prevention of osteoporosis. We'll talk more about that.

Calcium sources in your food can include dairy products—cheese, milk, yogurt have lots of calcium. Also, there are all the dark green leafy vegetables—spinach, chard, mustard greens, collared greens, romaine lettuce, and cabbage. Also, nuts and seeds—especially sesame seeds—beans, tofu, orange juice—which is often fortified with calcium—and even things like maple syrup. There are lots of ways to get calcium in your diet. This is one of the supplements that may be useful in certain groups of people.

Fiber—fiber is really what we call "roughage." It's basically the indigestible plant-food part that creates bulk in our digestive system. It absorbs water, which is a good thing because it keeps your bowels soft. It promotes easy defecation. It aids, we think, in getting rid of toxic wastes. It really is necessary, in some amount, for good digestive health. The name Denis Burkitt—who was a British epidemiologist, worked in Africa several decades ago—he noted that the local people ate whole grains rather than milled grains. They ate almost no processed food; lots of bulk and lots of fiber was in their diet. What he noticed was that they had almost no colon cancer, almost no diverticulitis, no appendicitis, and very little cardiovascular disease. They had, in general, about one or more large bulky stools a day. They weren't constipated. His theory is that, in the constipated society—which was actually very prevalent in Europe and the United States when he was overseas—led to a lot of the diseases of our digestive system because the toxins and the things we're trying to get rid of, the wastes, sit in contact with our colon longer. A lot of this is getting called into question now, but it doesn't hurt to look at that aspect and then see what we really need in fiber.

There is a little soft evidence that it might benefit protection from heart disease. Lowering total cholesterol is probably something that is real. It may decrease the risk of colon cancer and breast cancer. It may reduce blood sugar in diabetics. There's been a bit of debate about some of the benefits. But, right now, I think we should err on the side of plenty of fiber in our diets which we don't usually get in this country. I think this will improve bowel health. It tends to be more of a problem in the elderly as the colon loses its ability to pump. The muscular walls get a little dilated and weaker. This is made worse by laxatives and enemas. I'll get to that a lot later in the course.

What I recommend for you is to use fiber supplements if you're not getting enough fiber in your diet so that you are having at least one normal soft bowel movement a day. The way I do it is I get psyllium husks, either powdered or whole—I prefer them powdered—but you can also get this as over-the-counter drugs that are things like Metamucil. However, most of the ones that are already prepared have extra sugar and things you don't need. They're also expensive. You can go to a health food store and get some powdered psyllium for about a quarter of the price. I prepare it with berry juices—delicious grape juice, or other kinds of juices—stir it up into a frappe and have an evening smoothie. It's very palatable and the berries are adding another way to get in some antioxidant content. There's no correct dose. It's somewhere about a tablespoon a night for most people, but you have to figure it out. You'll know what's right when you take it in the evening and 12 hours later, you get the desired result. You'll be able to manipulate your own dose and see what works for you. It can be very consistent. It also adds a high satiety factor. It fills you up a bit, so people who want to cut calories sometimes take this before they sit down to dinner.

This brings us also to the area of herbal supplements. These are the supplements derived from plants. They're very, very popular. There are a lot of common ones in widespread use today. Some of the ones you hear about are ginkgo biloba, ginseng, and Echinacea—a lot of promoted benefits and very little science. For example, one of the most popular used ones is ginkgo biloba. It is touted to improve brain function based on increasing blood flow to the brain. There is no evidence of its effect, especially if the blood flow is normal, if that's not a problem. It does have some toxicity because it can increase the risk of bleeding disorders. Ginseng is very, very popular. It's been touted to improve energy levels and increase sexual performance. But, again, there's almost no science and a wide range of some toxic effects—maybe not serious ones, in most cases, but still annoying.

Echinacea has had a big, big market in this country. People believe it prevents infections, especially colds. Again, there is very little science. It has only a few side effects; it's probably very safe.

Ephedra, which was a weight loss medication, was proved to actually be lethal in a number of patients several years ago. It was finally removed from the market.

In the world of herbal supplements, in general, this is very early science. There is very scant literature and there are lots of problems. There are significant risks which do not always show up early. We don't find out about them because there's no reporting system in place to tell about the side effects. Additionally, there are so many compounds that it seems impossible that you could take them all without having some kind of a drug reaction or interaction and toxicity with other drugs. If you start getting into this herbal supplement cycle, there's really no end to it.

Let me talk a little bit about the caveats of supplements in general. Many legally sold dietary supplements have no FDA approval for safety or effectiveness. This is because they're treated as foods, not as drugs. Many other supplements have serious lethal potential when taken in large doses or with other supplements or other prescribed drugs. There's a lot of mixing and interactions that we really can't predict. For non-FDA approved drugs—for example, supplements and vitamins, as we mentioned, and food products—there's no reliable reporting system. We just don't know what's going on.

There were some statements in the NIH in 2006 which reported on dietary supplements in general. What they said was this: "The FDA has insufficient resources and legislative authority to require specific safety data from dietary supplement manufacturers or distributors, before or after their products are made available to the public. The constraints imposed on the FDA make it difficult for the health of the American public to be adequately protected." That's a chilling quote. We really have to take this into our own hands and provide our own responsibility.

In safety, the problem, for me, is the dose—which is very important—and content are not monitored by anybody, including the FDA. The pills may be especially hazardous from things like side effects, toxicity, and impurities. A full list of tainted pills and other details can be found on the FDA website. I would encourage you going there if you really want to use herbal supplements. Remember, again, just because something is natural doesn't mean it's safe and doesn't mean it's good for you. The unassailable conclusion of study after study is that you don't, and shouldn't, need to rely on supplements in place of whole food.

There are some criteria which you should look at before you use herbal supplements. In general, at the moment—with the exception of St. John's wort for mild depression, and valerian for sleeplessness—the majority of the herbal remedies have not been studied. There may be a problem for many, many years to come because you can't patent these. They are food based. They're available in nature, so nobody can own them. There's a very high cost to clinical studies—usually millions of dollars—so no manufacturer wants to pay for that because if they get good findings for their supplement, then anybody can immediately start selling it. The future may bring us new information, but for now, I'm really very skeptical and cautious about their uses.

Another big area which you can't have missed—if you go to any supermarket—are the commercially bottled or canned products, which again tout health benefits from added vitamins and other ingredients. There's little, if any, evidence that they do any good at all. There are oxygen containing drinks that absolutely have no benefit. They just take your money. Vitamin drinks have basically negligible value. Many additives, the fact that there are so many additives, make it hard to detect if a single one is dangerous. The more additives, the more risky it is. For example, they just found that, in the protein supplement that was one of the most popular ones used by bodybuilders, there had been several deaths which were caused by the supplement. This was a major protein supplement. It was taken off the market. But, nobody really knows what it was that caused the deaths yet. The content was an enormous amount of protein, but there could have been 50 or 100 different additives inside that provided the lethality. There are serious concerns, also, with the drinks high in sugar, caffeine, and other enhancing additives. People with cardiovascular disease or high blood pressure should be especially careful about these drinks.

In conclusion, although we can obtain most of the supplements through whole food, there are some supplements in pill form that can serve as valuable adjuncts in the general population and have valuable roles in nutrition if they're needed. I would have to say calcium and magnesium supplements, with or without vitamin D, are one of them—especially among women and older men where there's a concern for osteoporosis. Fish oils is another one I'm going to talk about in great detail at a later date. There are others that are plant based in the world of herbal supplements that might serve specific functions. So far, their science is scanty except for St. John's wort and valerian. The omega-3 fatty acids are continued as supplement and I want to give them adequate time. From here, we're going to move on to how we can get these vitamins and supplements in proper amounts from whole foods.

Whole Foods for Optimum Health
Lecture 15

It's a very common question I get—whether or not the intensity of the color in the food relates to the power of the various nutrients. The answer is no. Only a few of the many nutrients give a color to the food. Others that are still very important don't impart any color at all.

This lecture looks at some of the whole foods that are of particular value for us when we're aiming for optimum health. But remember, these are just a few of the hundreds of whole foods that should contribute to a healthy way of eating.

As mentioned earlier, **mitochondria** are organelles inside cells that are the home of energy production. Mitochondria are also the major producers of free radicals and become major targets of oxidative stress. One of the more controversial issues today is the role of the antioxidant polyphenol molecule resveratrol in reducing oxidative stress. Resveratrol is found in grape skins, grape juice, and red wine. In the laboratory, resveratrol supplements extend the lifespans of mice, but no reliable studies of its effects on humans have been performed. Another group of molecules called sirtuins have been implicated in the regulation of aging, transcription, apoptosis, and stress resistance, but again, research on sirtuins is in its infancy.

Polyphenols are organic chemicals that belong to a family of several thousand compounds referred to as flavonoids. They're found in large amounts in fruits, berries, pomegranates, grapes, wine,

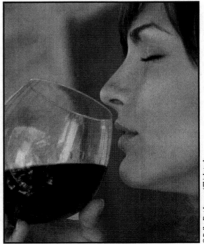

© Polka Dot Images/ Thinkstock.

Large amounts of polyphenols are found in grapes and red wine.

walnuts, olive oil, chocolate, cocoa, coffee, and tea. Their antioxidant properties can reduce the risk of cancer and cardiovascular diseases.

How do we get the benefits of these molecules that are in food without going into an area of unproven claims and possible risks? The answer is whole foods. There is a great deal of debate about eating organically grown foods versus eating foods that may have been treated with pesticides and other chemicals. My position is that these chemicals are very harmful to our health, especially to the health of children.

As a group, berries are packed full with beneficial nutrients, including resveratrol and the sirtuins, but note that nonorganic berries tend to be grown using many chemicals. Blackberries, raspberries, elderberries, strawberries, and açai berries all contain, among other compounds, anthocyanins, which are powerful antioxidants. They appear to inhibit cancer development by several mechanisms, including minimizing DNA damage. They also reduce inflammation, slow the growth of premalignant cells, and inhibit tumor angiogenesis (the growth of new blood vessels in tumors).

Phytochemicals, meaning those from plants, protect against breast, colon, and liver cancer in the laboratory. In apples, these anticancer properties are primarily concentrated in the peel, but again, choose organic if possible because pesticides tend to stick to the waxy skins of apples. Plums, both fresh and dried, are also high in antioxidants and are effective in neutralizing superoxide radicals, which result in oxidative stress. Concord grapes and grape juice offer the broadest range of polyphenols and the highest overall antioxidant concentration capacity.

Both allicin in garlic and curcumin in tumeric are antioxidants and anti-inflammatories. Recent studies suggest that allicin may reduce atherosclerosis and fat deposition in the blood vessels and improve lipoprotein balance.

Finally, **probiotics** are active bacteria found in yogurt and yogurt-like foods and are sold as supplements. Their active bacteria are good for you, but there's no evidence that these bacteria are any better than the bacteria that are already present in the colon. ■

mitochondria: The cell's powerhouses and the source of energy in the engines of the cell.

polyphenols: Common antioxidant molecules found in nature that may inhibit LDL oxidation and, thereby prevent arterial plaque formation.

probiotics: Active bacteria added to foods to promote digestive health; they can be found in yogurt.

Questions to Consider

1. What are anthocyanins? What is their function in the body? What is a food source for them?

2. What are the pros and cons of taking megadoses of a chemical, such as resveratrol?

Whole Foods for Optimum Health
Lecture 15—Transcript

Welcome back. Today, let's take a look at some of the whole foods that are of particular value for us when we're aiming for optimum health. Many of these you'll recognize because they have been discussed more and more in health literature, newspapers, and magazines. But, they may not yet be on your shopping list. Remember, these are just a few of hundreds and hundreds of whole foods that comprise a healthy way of eating.

First, let's search for antioxidants that are of proven value. There's a lot of discussion about antioxidants and what they are and why they matter in our diet. But, here, we're going to be talking about finding the valuable substances such as antioxidants, and others, in whole food rather than the supplements. One issue I want to mention right off the bat—and I'll repeat this more and more as it becomes clear why it's so important in our search— most of the time, getting your vital nutrients from whole foods will make it much less likely that you're going to get a toxic overdose. The same cannot be said of supplements, such as pills or liquids. There may be exceptions, but that would require such an unbalanced diet that it really shouldn't be a problem for most of you. In general, getting all your nutrition from whole foods is, in the long run, the safest strategy. It's a major theme throughout the course.

Let's talk about, quickly, oxidative stress and mitochondrial dysfunction which we looked at a little bit in the beginning. Remember, the mitochondria are the powerhouses of our cells. They're the tiny little organs, or organelles, inside cells, that are the home of energy production. Mitochondria are also the major producers of free radicals during the energy process. They become the major target themselves of oxidative damage. That word, "oxidative stress," is defined as the elevation of free radicals beyond what the body's capability is to neutralize them. They are reactive oxygen molecules and we're trying to get them back to normal safe levels. It's very, very vague. It's not easily measured as a clinical entity. There's no test for them, really, that's of significance. We can't tell, then, what the levels are of the free radicals or give them a number or define oxidative stress by what's safe and how many free radicals. But, we can look at the results of the damage and we can get very soft estimates.

Excessive oxidative stress does damage to the cells and tissues, and specifically the mitochondria, the cell membranes which hold the cell together and are kind of like the spacesuit I talked about for our whole body. It damages DNA, it damages proteins, and fats. The search is to find molecules that bring these back to normal. We don't want to eliminate them because we need some of them as useful tools in fighting other threats.

One of the newer and most controversial issues today is the role of an antioxidant polyphenol molecule called "resveratrol." Resveratrol is produced by plants in response to their own stress. It's found in grape skins, grape juice, and especially in red wine. In the laboratory, it extends the life of non-mammalian organisms. Also in the laboratory, it improves the metabolic profile and the lifespan of the mice that are fed diets high in fat. Remember, mice don't usually eat high-fat diets in nature, so this gets very artificial. But, mice fed very high doses of resveratrol and fed these high-fat diets had survival rates similar to control mice on a normal diet. It also enhanced the performance of the mice in motor skill testing. But, with equivalent doses, the average human would need to drink about 100 to 1,000 bottles of red wine a day to get the same resveratrol levels as the mice did in this study.

Supplements of resveratrol are available. My worry is that the doses are not standardized. The side effects have not yet been well studied in humans. There's enormous pharmacological dosing here. Remember I talked to you about physiologic doses and pharmacologic doses—what we get naturally in nature and these big doses that are way out of proportion. There is no science on the side effects or the toxicity of these huge doses over the long term. Essentially, there've been no human studies that we can rely on. It's going to be a very long time before there are any because, in order to prove what these people are trying to prove, you would need studies that go on for decades to see if they prolong life. Right now, we don't have that.

There's another group of molecules called "sirtuins." This is an acronym for silent information regulator proteins and there's a whole group of them. They're also found in the skins of dark-colored grapes, other vegetables, and fruits. They regulate important biologic pathways in many, many organisms from bacteria up through some of the more evolved organisms. They have been implicated in the regulation of aging, of transcription—remember, that's the copying of DNA information—apoptosis, the scheduled cell suicide, and stress resistance. It's a very important molecule. They regulate metabolic processes and cell defenses. There might be a role, in the future, for these sirtuin in lifespan prolongation in mammals. But, we don't know yet. It's very, very early. This is really in its infancy. Resveratrol is also thought to be a sirtuin activator and this is another benefit that may prove out in time. Right now, I don't know of any data that these chemicals, taken as supplements, will lengthen human life or retard aging.

There's a very real question in my mind of the possible toxic effects of megadosing. They have not been tested in human clinical trials. Remember, Phase 1 trials always are looking for the safety first. We don't have the results of those trials yet. We have no reliable safety data. I know lots of people who take these drugs. I don't and my family doesn't.

Let's move on and look at polyphenols. As we talked about in our last lecture, polyphenols are one of the organic chemicals among several thousand compounds referred to as "flavonoids." They're found in very large amounts in fruits, berries, pomegranates, grapes, wine, walnuts, olive oil, and in beverages such as chocolate, cocoa, coffee, and tea. The highest level of most of these chemicals is generally in the peel of the fruit. In others, they're in the pulp. You should eat both of these if you possibly can—if it's safe to eat the skin, which it isn't always. Their antioxidant properties can reduce the risk of both cancer and cardiovascular diseases. Remember, when we go from the laboratory to humans, we don't always go to these prospective studies right away because we don't have them. But, we can look at those societies we mentioned before who have diets rich with these fruits and vegetables and they've been our test case. These are the places where people have lived long, long lives, and been very healthy right into old age. That experiment has been done out in the real world.

Let me make a short digression now about the color of foods. It's a very common question I get—whether or not the intensity of the color in the food relates to the power of the various nutrients. The answer is no. Only a few of the many nutrients give a color to the food. Others that are still very important don't impart any color at all. Many, many nutrients are absolutely colorless just like water. Within groups like grapes, apples, or onions, separate groups, and others, the color is not a good guideline for you to look at for nutrient value. One warning is that, in processed foods—which are going to be kind of the whipping boy for me—the color may be processed right out with the nutrients. In what the manufacturer does to the food, the color is lost and the nutrients are lost. Then, what they do is they put in artificial colors because they've lost all the nutrients that have the color. For me, this is a particular nightmare. I happen to be very sensitive to artificial food dyes. This is the first thing I look for whenever I buy any food. Many people are affected by this. I'll talk to that later.

How do we get the benefits of these molecules that are in the food without going into an area of unproven benefits and possible risks? The answer is whole foods. I want to talk to the whole issue of organic food and choices you have in buying organic or not organic food. It's a great deal of research being done by the government, non-governmental agencies, private and corporate sectors, and individual farmers about the benefits of organic versus non-organic foods. The data as to the upside of eating organically grown foods versus the downside of eating foods that may have been raised with pesticides, insecticides, and other chemicals is a very, very hot debate. It's a very important one in my opinion. This is one of those areas where I said I would tell you where there's science, what is still under investigation, and where I personally stand. In this case, I've taken a very strong position.

I've been growing some of my own food since medical school, starting with a little tomato plant in my windowsill. It was really pathetic, this little wilted plant that I now look back on in a dirty window in the middle of New York City. But, with a lot of care, it provided me ultimately with one whole salad full of cherry tomatoes. It started me on a whole growing career with my own food as the product. Since then, I've moved from bigger pots out in the backyard growing vegetables to a vegetable garden that was about as big as this table—maybe two by four feet—and then to bigger farms when we lived in New Zealand. Now, in Montana, we have our own greenhouse and a very large garden. Growing some portion of my own food has continued to be very, very important for me—and my whole family—for lots of reasons.

For over 40 years, I've grown completely organic, pesticide and chemical free fruits and vegetables. I know what those chemicals can do. They smell terrible and they feel terrible when you actually touch them. The ones that are in these pesticides and insecticides are very, very harmful to our health. They are not good for us, period. They're especially bad for children because their bodies are growing, their cells are turning over fast, and the dose is much, much higher in a 30 or 40 pound child than in a 160 pound adult. Given the same exposure, the child is getting way higher doses.

Some of the research is still under debate—there are arguments on either side and there are statistics about acceptable limits that are now being negotiated by the food industry. In the meantime, my family chooses to eat as much organic produce as we can possibly get. We've done this for many, many years. It's one area where I think—I'm personally convinced—that it serves our health. I think, if you look at it, it should be a place you look to for changing if you're not already eating organic foods. As a medical professional and someone interested in this whole area, and then at the same time as a consumer of lots of fruits—and probably not enough vegetables according to my wife—having raised a family with the healthiest food that we can provide really matters to me. I hope it'll start to matter to you. Again, looking back at those societies and the people who eat diets high in fruits and vegetables, they have significantly lower cancer rates, they live longer lives, and they're healthier well into old age.

Now let's take a look at those power foods and be specific in what they might do for us. First of all, there are the berries. As a group, these are just packed full with multiple beneficial nutrients. The berries are supercharged with ingredients and molecules including resveratrol and the sirtuins. Just as a warning, as an aside—in general, avoid eating berries that are not organic. Non-organic berries tend to be grown using many, many chemicals. Some of the chemicals can be washed off the surface but not all of them. Some of the foods that tend to be heavy in pesticides and chemicals include—and these are the ones you should really look for organic sources of—peaches, apples, sweet bell peppers, celery, nectarines, cherries especially, kale, lettuce, grapes—which tend to be imported out of season and tend to have a lot of pesticides on them—carrots, and pears. You probably want to buy those organically if you can, or maybe avoid them if you cannot.

Research done on things like blackberries, both black and red raspberries, elderberries, and strawberries, strongly suggest that they are really potent health producing fruits. There's a new player on the scene in the last few years called the açai berry, grown primarily in South America, and touted as the new super food. It may be. We don't have any scientific data yet. It's way too early, but it is packed full of a lot of nutrients just like the other berries. Right now, it's a $100 million per year industry. It probably should go into the mix of the many berries you want to eat or the juices you want to drink. There's no science to support it as a massive use, for example, in juices or extracts, but it's a good thing to have in the mix.

All these berries also contain other compounds that are healthy for us. This includes anthocyanins. "Anthos" means flower and "cyanin" means blue. These are the blue flowers that were first seen in these berries and they give the berries their color. They belong to a big, big parent class of flavonoids. The anthocyanins are also very, very powerful antioxidants. Their antioxidant property is passed onto us when we eat the fruit, it's not destroyed. In lab experiments, at least, it suggests that their health effects of these berries give us protection against cancer, some aspects of aging, inflammation—which tends to be one of the real problems in cell damage—diabetes, and some neurological and brain diseases. But, we don't have long-term controlled studies yet. It's still in its infancy. We have to look back to the societies that eat a lot of these foods and see that they're doing very, very well.

As we discussed in some of the earlier lectures, the nutritional studies in humans are very, very difficult. They tend to be hugely expensive, talking millions of dollars. They don't benefit the person who funds the study because all these products and fruits can't be patented. The people who spend the money may likely not benefit from it. They're very hard to control because of the inaccuracy because of personal dietary diaries. We don't know also what else that person may be eating that they don't remember they're eating. Also, there are variations in the nutritional content of even the same food groups. Some of the lab findings are interesting; they may or may not apply to us in the real world, we'll have to see.

Anthocyanins appear to inhibit cancer development by several mechanisms. First, they minimize DNA damage. Remember that damage to DNA is very important in the development of cancer. What happens is that the replication of DNA into the next generation of cells may get misinformation passed along. This is where we go down the line of incorrect information possibly leading to mutations that cause cancer. These anthocyanins may stop that from happening.

They also reduce inflammation which, besides giving you things like arthritis and joint pain, is also a precursor to some cancers. For example, hepatitis, inflammation of the liver, around the world, can be a precursor over a lifetime to developing liver cancer. They slow the growth of premalignant cells which his very important. They may promote apoptosis, the programmed cell suicide so that in damaged cells that have the wrong information, these chemicals may prevent them from being replicated and may actually cause them to be killed. They inhibit tumor angiogenesis—this is a word we haven't come across before—and slow or halt the growth of cancer cells because cancer cells need blood vessels. That's what angiogenesis is, the ingrowth of new blood vessels. These molecules may stop that. These are all laboratory experiments. We call that *in vitro*, meaning in glass, as opposed to *in vivo* meaning in real life.

Again, my bias would be to stick with the whole fruit and juice and not go to the supplements. Also, they taste good—much better than capsules. They have lots of chemicals not included in the supplements, chemicals that are already in the fruit. This may take decades to define—to look at and see what result they have in aiding other chemicals that we're eating. We don't want to wait decades for information to see when some of these supplements might benefit us. We have the healthy food right here and we know they work. You have some choices. I know sometimes it's difficult to find fresh fruit that doesn't have pesticide or insecticide contamination. When fresh berries are out of season—and they tend to be more expensive then—or they're not available at all organically, try frozen berries. They don't spoil, they're generally available all year round, and they're generally less expensive than fresh berries because they've been bought at a time when there's a lot of supply. Also, you can buy them when they're in season. They're less expensive and then freeze them yourself. It's very easy to do. Then, you've got it and you know where it came from. They're great in shakes and smoothies and they do maintain most of their nutrients in the frozen state.

Now, more on some great power foods. There are lots of them that we can get out there that are delicious and they'll give you a lot of benefit. First of all are apples. We think the anticancer properties are primarily concentrated in the peel. You should therefore be very cognizant of where your apples come from. They need to be organic if possible. Phytochemicals, meaning those chemicals that are from the plant, protect against breast cancer, colon cancer, and liver cancer in the laboratory. Remember, pesticides tend to stick to the waxy skins of apples, something that's often put on them also to protect them. Therefore, you want to be able to wash them off whenever you can. It's better to get organic, but if you have to buy the inorganic, make sure you wash them. It's very important. There are special soaps that are more effective that you can buy in the supermarkets to get the waxiness off and chemicals off.

Plums are a new player actually. People are now recognizing that plums—both in the fresh version such as plums themselves, and in the dried version, the prunes—are very, very high in antioxidants as well as phenols. They're very effective in neutralizing what we call the "superoxide radicals," those free radicals that tend to oxidize and give us oxidative stress. They prevent some oxygen-based damage to fats in our neurons. Remember, fats insulate neurons and play a very important part in normal neuron function and brain function. Add those to your fruit-weapons quiver. They're very important.

Concord grapes and grape juice—this is one of my favorite groups. They top the list of the broadest range of polyphenols and the highest overall antioxidant concentration capacity. In my opinion, why not use the grape juice version instead of the wine version? There's more resveratrol and some other beneficial chemicals in wine than grape juice. But, remember, then you're taking the alcohol. We're going to talk a lot more about alcohol later. But, remember now that one of the things we do know is that women—even when they only take a small amount of alcohol in the diet—stepwise increase their risk of breast cancer with each level of alcohol intake. They can get very nearly the same nutrition from grape juice as they could from wine, without the alcohol risk.

What I try to do with all these berries is, I combine as many different compounds by combining as many different juices as I can. I'll go out and buy some blueberry juice, pomegranate, açai, concord grape, and so on, get them home and mix them all into one container. I keep them in the refrigerator, and use that as a drink throughout the day. I try to stick to sources that are 100% juice. You can see that on the label, even if it's from concentrate. I try to make sure they're always organic. I don't usually go for what are labelled "nectars" or "mixtures" of juices because usually—if you look on what they'll often label as an antioxidant mix—if you look on the back, you'll often see the first ingredient is water and then some juices that may not be so good, and then some added sugar, and little bits of the juices you're after. Go and get the 100% juice and mix those. You'll get more bang for your buck. It also tastes better to me when they're mixed but that's a personal decision. Don't forget about the psyllium berry juice smoothie. You can mix all your fiber in there and get a terrific shot of antioxidants and enough fiber.

Garlic, one of my favorite, favorite foods—I grow a lot of organic garlic. I have for many, many years. There's a whole different chemistry from the berries. Garlic contains an organic flavor compound called "allicin." It's a very, very potent antioxidant. When it decomposes, it generates something called "sulfenic acid." That too is an even more powerful antioxidant. The reaction between free radicals and sulfenic acid is instantaneous. No other compound, natural or synthetic, responds as fast as this antioxidant.

Recent studies suggest that allicin might do a lot of things. It seems to reduce atherosclerosis and fat deposition in your vessels so it helps with hardening of the arteries. It improves that lipoprotein balance, the HDL that you want to go up and the LDL/VLDL proteins that you want to go down. It possesses some anti-clotting activity that makes it rather good in things like stroke and some kinds of heart attacks. It promotes anti-inflammatory activity, which we now know is a good thing, and it increases antioxidant activity of other molecules. There's almost no downside. It's delicious and it's really easy to grow. It's hard not to be a successful garlic grower.

Let's quickly take a look at some more good foods. A new player now is tumeric which is a spice that's been used in Asia and India for a long time. It's used in curries and in mustard. Its active component is curcumin. It's an antioxidant, anti-inflammatory. It has effects on more than 700 genes. It inhibits both the activity and the making of cyclooxgenase-2. Remember,

COX-2, the COX-2 inhibitors were terrific. Celebrex was one of them. Unfortunately, although they gave terrific results with getting joint pain under control, they had other side effects. First, taken off the market, now back with a lot of warnings. You can get this in tumeric. Low-toxicity food and some people are trying to put it again into a supplemental extract, we don't know if that works at all. At this point, it's just more good food that'll support your health.

Teas are another area that interest me. True teas come from the *Camellia sinensis*, a Chinese camellia—very, very rich in polyphenol. The main ingredient is epigallocatechin gallate, EGCG, a highly-powerful antioxidant. Herbal teas don't fall into this category. They may have specific medicinal properties, but they're not true teas. They generally don't have any EGCG. The major problem, in the science, is that the proven levels of effective active ingredients in the tea which positively affect your health are in amounts that would require drinking dozens of cups a day. Then that brings in too much caffeine, not enough benefit. The take away is that, while green teas are probably good for you, don't go overboard. Drink them if you enjoy them.

Finally, there are probiotics which are yogurt-like substances that are sold as supplements. They have active bacteria which are good for you. But, there's really no evidence that these bacteria—which are supposed to improve the bacteria in your colon— are really any better than the bacteria that are already there. They might be useful in patients who've had their own bacteria wiped out by antibiotics, but other than that, they sound good. They probably don't have a downside, but the science has not kept up with the promotions of the advertising companies.

There are many, many wonderful whole foods, chock-full of naturally occurring vitamins and supplements. A whole and varied diet should provide most people with all of their nutritional needs. Next time, we'll move on to other powerful foods that often get a bad rap—some good, healthy fat.

The Good Fats
Lecture 16

> Read the labels. Look for the sources. Ask good questions. Become an educated consumer. ... A lot of the changes have occurred because of people like you going out and demanding cleaner, safer food and good knowledge of the sources.

According to general dietary recommendations, your total fat intake should be kept below about 30 percent of your daily calories. In a 2,000-calorie diet, that would mean less than about 650 calories of fat. Of that fat, less than half of it should be saturated fat.

Fatty acids are **organic** acids composed of a chain of carbons and multiple hydrogens attached to those carbons. Unsaturated fats break down into monounsaturated and polyunsaturated fats. The latter include an important group called omega fatty acids. The omega-3 fatty acid group is found in coldwater fish, such as herring, salmon, mackerel, tuna, and so on. High consumption of the omega-3s has proven positive effects, particularly with regard to cardiovascular disease. A small amount of **omega-6 fatty acids** in the diet also promotes good health, but an overabundance is unhealthy. Omega-6s are found in red meat and various vegetable oils.

In general, both groups—the omega-3s and the omega-6s—have positive effects on health if eaten in the right proportions. Most scientists believe that human beings evolved and prospered on a diet with a 1-to-1 ratio of omega-6s to omega-3s. Our modern diet tends to have a ratio of about 15 to 1. We have a huge excess of omega-6 fatty acids in our diet, primarily because of processed foods. The maximum healthy ratio is probably less than 4 to 1.

Studies show that the 4-to-1 ratio or below yielded about a 70 percent decrease in total mortality from cardiovascular disease over higher ratios. The omega-3 fatty acids from fish or fish oil supplements significantly decreased blood triglyceride levels, which are associated with heart disease. Omega-3s may also prevent age-related macular degeneration, reduce joint tenderness in patients with rheumatoid arthritis, reduce cognitive decline and dementias, and have many other positive effects. The omega-6 fatty acids, in low or normal levels, positively affect brain function, body growth and development in the young, and many functions in the clotting system. But high levels of omega-6 are associated with heart attacks, strokes, arthritis, and even mood disorders.

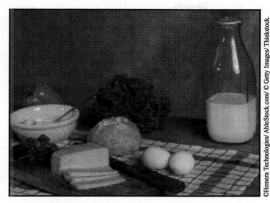

Saturated fatty acids come mainly from sausage, bacon, cakes and cookies, chocolate, cheese, eggs, and milk. If possible, replace **saturated fats** with monounsaturated

Eggs, milk, and cheese are sources of saturated fats.

fats, such as olive oil, nuts, avocados, and so on. These will decrease LDL cholesterol and triglycerides and maintain high HDL cholesterol.

Polyunsaturated fats can be found in vegetable oils, coldwater fish, nuts of all kinds, and sunflower seeds. Cross-cultural studies show that inhabitants of the countries that surround the Mediterranean seem to gain some protection against heart disease from the large quantities of monounsaturated fats they consume in their normal diet. Eating a handful of mixed nuts daily has also been shown to reduce symptoms of heart disease.

Remember, the quality of the fat is more important than the total fat in the diet. When you can, substitute vegetable fats for animal fats. Substitute fish proteins for animal proteins. Replace whole milk with skim milk or 2 percent milk. Eliminate solid margarine, commercially baked goods, and deep-fried and fast foods to reduce the consumption of trans-fatty acids. ■

omega-3 fatty acids: Highly unsaturated fats needed for the production of hormone-like compounds known as prostaglandins.

organic: Biologic compounds or molecules found in nature that have a carbon base; also, plant and animal products defined by a particular method of farming that uses no chemical pesticides and no chemical fertilizers.

saturated fats: Long carbon–fatty acid chains that have no double bond because the whole molecule is saturated with hydrogen ions.

1. Define monounsaturated, polyunsaturated, and saturated fats. How do they each affect health in humans? In what food sources would you find these fats?

2. What are some ways you can increase the good fats and reduce the bad fats in your diet?

The Good Fats
Lecture 16—Transcript

Welcome back. Today, I want to look at another group of whole foods that have potential for maximizing health and well-being. This is a group of foods that are greatly misunderstood, the good fats. Even the role of total dietary fat in obesity is still misunderstood and uncertain. All fats are just not created equal. Beginning with the general dietary recommendations—which you can follow easily—your total fat intake should be kept below about 30 percent of your daily calories. In a 2,000 calorie diet, which is average in this country, that would mean less than about 650 calories of fat. Of that fat, less than half of it should be saturated fat, in fact, as little as possible. I want to review the vocabulary and some of the essential chemistry of the fats once again because we're going to talk about it a lot.

Fatty acids are organic acids with up to about 26 carbons, long chain of carbons, and lots of hydrogen attached to those carbons. These are the three fatty acids I pointed to earlier that are hanging off the glycerine molecule like the capital letter "E." They're saturated fats where all the hydrogen places possible for attachment to the carbon are taken. They're generally solid at room temperature. They're generally not good for you.

Then there are the unsaturated fats which have some carbon atoms that lack the full complement of hydrogen. They tend to be liquid at room temperature. They're good for the fish and they're good for us. This group breaks itself down into the monounsaturated fats, which have just one carbon with an empty slot for its hydrogen, and then the polyunsaturated fats which have more than one carbon with empty slots. These are also liquid at room temperature and even very low temperatures beyond room temperature.

Polyunsaturated fats—which you'll see referred to as "PUFA" in the literature—include an important group which we call the "omega fatty acids." "Omega" just refers to structure, where things are placed on the molecule. It's not function, so it's important to the chemists, but really not to us. One group of the polyunsaturated fatty acids, the PUFAs, is a kind of fatty acid we call "essential." It cannot be synthesized by the body like the essential amino acids.

They're divided into several categories, but two of the important ones are the omega-3 and the omega-6 fatty acids. We'll start with the omega-3s. These are one of the good fats, by and large. I'll give you the caveats or the warnings in a minute. Ideally, we need to find more ways to incorporate these into our diets. This is one place where I have to back off my other statement and say that supplementation may make sense for some of us. Let's see what they are, how they work, and what you might do to get them into your diet.

First, there's the omega-3 fatty acid group. These include—and I want to say the names because you're going to hear them over and over again—alpha linoleic acid, or ALA; eicosapentaenoic acid, EPA; and docosahexaenoic acid, DHA. The body can convert any one of these omega-3s into another omega-3. But, they can't convert them into the next group we'll talk about which is the omega-6 group. You'll find these fatty acids in large quantities in fatty cold-water fish such as herring, salmon, mackerel, tuna, halibut, cod, and several others. These fish need fats, again, as I mentioned before, that stay liquid at low temperatures so they don't solidify while they're trying to swim. There are strong health benefits when we eat these fish in our diet in recommended amounts. They're of extra value when they also replace some of the saturated fats or even trans-fats in our diet, because more fish meals probably mean you're eating fewer meat meals. In fact, it's hard for me to decide whether it's the fish meals that we consume every week that are the benefit entirely in themselves, or is it combined with the fact that each fish meal replaces a meat meal which may be high in saturated fats? I don't know the answer and I don't think it matters. It's good to eat lots of fish. It's probably both.

High consumption of the omega-3s has proven impacts on life. Strong evidence comes from studies on both fish in the diet and now also from fish oil supplements. When it comes to cardiovascular disease which is, after all, the biggest killer, eating omega-3 fatty acids—both fish and fish oil or either/or—decreases the all-cause mortality. This includes heart attacks, sudden cardiac death of any kind, and other heart-related conditions that cause death-like rhythm disturbances.

The other group of fatty acids, the omega-6 fatty acids, has a little more subtlety in what we have to look for. Overall, a small amount of the omega-

6s in our diets promotes good health. It's the overabundance that's unhealthy. Omega-6s include some acids like linoleic acid, LA—remember the other one in the omega-3s was alpha linoleic acid. This is different. There is also arachidonic acid. Again, the body can convert one of these acids in the O-6s to the other acid and back and forth. But, they too can't go and be converted into the omega-3s. This is why we're going to have to select carefully which we put into our body because our body can't balance it for us. They generally are part of a healthy regimen for the heart. You can get omega-6s from red meat, vegetable oils, corn oil, cottonseed oil, peanut oil, safflower oil, soy bean oil—starts to sound familiar. They're a lot of our foods. It's very, very common in processed foods. We have no shortage of the sixes, and that's the problem.

In general, both groups—the O-3s and the O-6s—have positive effects on health if they're given in the right proportions or if they're eaten in the right proportions. The key in the sentence is "the right proportions." The O-3s tend to be very, very anti-inflammatory. When inflammation in excess, like in arthritis or in our arteries, is the problem, you get good benefit from the omega-3s. The omega-6s tend to be proinflammatory. Inflammation is a good thing—it's a body defense—in limited amounts. Again, we're back to proportion. The ratio of the O-6 to the O-3 appears to be what's most important with these two groups. It's absolutely critical to health. Most scientists believe that human beings evolved and prospered, did very well, on a diet—and now we're talking over hundreds of thousands of years—of a one-to-one ratio, the same amount of omega-6s as the omega-3 polyunsaturated fatty acids.

Interest in this really started when they studied the omegas. This is because they found that there were very low rates of coronary artery heart disease among some Greenland Inuits, or Eskimos, who ate very, very large amounts of very fatty seafood. This was surprising at the time. What they found in the Inuit diet was that the ratio of omega-6 to omega-3 was about two-and-a-half to one and maybe up to six to one in favor of the omega-6s. Compare that to our diet where the ratio is 15 to one. We have 15 times as much omega-6 as omega-3. That's a huge difference. That's because we have a deficiency of the omega-3 fatty acids in our modern diet. We have a huge excess of omega-6 fatty acids in our modern diet, and especially in those processed foods.

The problem is, how do we get the right ratio? The best estimate about the maximum healthy ratio is probably that it should be less than four to one of the omega-6s to the omega-3s. It's hard for us to approach that one-to-one ratio that we had when we were walking on our knuckles, but four to one is probably pretty good. The studies regarding the O-6 to O-3 ratios are very interesting. The four-to-one ratio or below yielded about a 70 percent decrease in total mortality from cardiovascular disease over the higher ratios that we usually find in our diet. The omega-3 fatty acids from fish or from fish oil supplements, which included EPA and DHA, significantly decreased blood triglyceride levels. Remember, high triglycerides are associated with heart disease. The omega-3s reduced the possibility of fatal and non-fatal heart attacks. They reduced sudden death. They reduced death from any cause in patients who had prior heart attacks. They reduced vascular inflammation which we are now, again, beginning to think is the key to reducing heart attacks. In other words, the narrowing that you get from just the atherosclerosis may be made worse, more narrow, in our vessels, by the added inflammation. It also may prevent age-related macular degeneration which is a cause of blindness, and a great deal of unhappiness in the elderly.

It has impacts on other conditions. There's reduced joint tenderness in patients with rheumatoid arthritis, so that's the anti-inflammatory effect. Cognitive decline and dementias are reduced possibly from, again, anti-inflammatory effects in the brain. Depression is reduced. Asthma is reduced. There are positive effects on stroke and cancer—in other words, reductions. These are the same as with cardiovascular disease, but a little bit lower magnitude. The omega-6 fatty acids, in low or normal levels, will positively affect brain function, normal body growth and development in the young, and many, many functions in the complex clotting system. We have a clotting system that has many, many steps, and every one of those has to be perfect. But, in high levels of the omega-6, you get increases instead—of heart attack, strokes of the thrombotic type which means clotting, arrhythmias, arthritis, osteoporosis, all kinds of inflammation, and even mood disorders. The conclusions on the omegas in the diet—there are many, major benefits from getting many, many more omega-3s and really limiting our omega-6s in the usual Western diet.

There was a Harvard School of Public Health study that showed the low omega-3 intake ranked as the sixth biggest killer in the United States when linked to the diseases that it may be associated with. This was implicated in about 84,000 preventable deaths. Just out of interest, numbers one to five ahead of this were tobacco, of course, high blood pressure, obesity, physical inactivity, and a high salt intake. In this study, the lowest risk came with consumption of more than about 250 milligrams of the omega-3s. The recommendations worldwide are very variable. They talk about a total intake of between 500 and 1,000 milligrams a day for optimal health.

You can get that with fish and other foods and not ever have to go to a supplement. For example, a 3.5 ounce serving of salmon has about somewhere between 1,200 milligrams or 2,300 milligrams, depending on the source of the salmon. You don't have to go out and catch a 65 pound king salmon. You can go and get a small 3 ounce filet of salmon a few times a week and get all you need. It's probably best to get it from those coldwater fish, or you can get it from nuts or flax. Otherwise, if you just can't get this into your diet, supplements will do the job. You do want to remember, however, that supplements of fish oil need to come from clean sources where the oil is pure and fresh.

Let's turn now to the coldwater fish and some of their fats and see how the choice of fish species and preparing the food—cooking—really matters. There was a large scale study of 900 patients—again, this is a pretty good sized study. What they found was that, at first, total fish consumption didn't seem to strongly correlate with EPA and DH levels in the patients' bloods. When they looked carefully at the study, they realized that a lot of these people were frying their fish, deep frying them in oil. What they needed was to get rid of the fried fish in the study and start again. They wanted to replace it with non-fried fish. They found that, once they did that, they found the differences for the healthy oils. The frying at very high temperatures seemed to destroy some of the omega-3s so they just weren't getting what they thought they were getting. Cooking at lower temperatures and shorter cooking time is preferable. You can cook these fish, for example, in broth or you can poach them. But, you don't need to fry them or cook them at high temperatures.

You should try to select fish that are high in the omega-3s. Once again, those include wild cod, Pacific salmon, scallops which I love, shrimp which I also love, cod, tuna, herring, sardines—lots of choices, lots of delicious available fish. We then have to get into the issue of farm fish versus wild caught fish. Here's where I do have a strong preference just the way I did on organic. You can't really get organic fish. It's not possible to control their environment that much, but I always go for the wild caught species if I can. I really believe it's important to focus on eating wild fish as much as we can. For me, it's because of, primarily, the chemicals, additives, and antibiotics that are used in farm salmon and many, many other farmed fish. These additives also get out into the environment, for example, like the open ocean. They affect other fish that may be nearby.

Farm salmon are also commonly fed food dyes to make their meat look pinker or more red, because much of the farm fish looks very pale. If you'll just look at most of the labels on smoked salmon from farmed species, you'll see, on the back, that they have chemical food dyes in the majority of them. You have to look carefully to get rid of that. This adds nothing to the nutritional value of the salmon, but it increases some of the dangers that are being recognized as associated with artificial dyes. You'd be amazed about how much information there is available, especially if you have the access to smaller butchers, fish stores, seafood shops, other local stores, and farmers markets. Also, today, I think, in most places, you can go and look to the managers of major supermarkets. They'll be very interested in hearing what you have to say and sharing information. They're usually quite knowledgeable. You just have to ask after them and pin them down the first few times.

Read the labels. Look for the sources. Ask good questions. Become an educated consumer. Be the squeaky wheel and keep after your people so you know the sources, until you get the information you want. A lot of the changes have occurred because of people like you going out and demanding cleaner, safer food, and good knowledge of the sources. It can happen.

We should aim at increasing our omega-3 and decreasing our omega-6 fatty acids in our diet and at least get closer to that one-to-one ratio. We should just aspire to get closer to that than this 15-to-1 ratio we're getting now. Avoid huge overdoses of the omegas, especially the supplements. It's easy to pop a few extra pills and you are then risking internal bleeding or a synergy, especially if you're on anticoagulant medications. These reduce blood clotting and that could get out of hand. Again, I'd like to see you get it from fish. But, be careful when you're using the supplements. They can help you, but you have to know what you're doing.

Saturated fatty acids are a problem for us. They come mainly from animal fats, sausages, bacon—all delicious things—cakes and cookies which I also love, chocolate, dairy, cheese, eggs, and milk—everything we've grown up loving. There is a straight line relationship between coronary heart disease events of a bad kind, and total serum cholesterol. Saturated fats can be converted and they raise the total serum cholesterol in humans. The monounsaturated fats are very, very important. If you can replace your saturated fats with the monounsaturated fats such as olive oil—which is delicious—nuts, avocado, and so on, they will decrease your LDL cholesterol, the bad guys, and the triglycerides, which are bad. They maintain your high HDL cholesterol, which is good. They decrease the oxidation of LDL cholesterol which is bad for you, too. The oxidized cholesterol is bad. The oxidation exacerbates atherosclerosis, meaning it makes it worse. This may prevent thrombosis by keeping away from that. This is the final event in myocardial infarction, or heart attack, when the vessels get narrow, narrow, narrow. Finally, the last thing that happens is blood clots form. The omegas in the natural foods can prevent that from happening. You can substitute, for example, the butter that we love to put on our bread—I certainly love it—with a little olive oil, salt, and pepper. Put that on your bread instead—another way of getting olive oil into your diet.

The polyunsaturated fats—remember that the omega fatty acids are a large part of this group in human nutrition and health. You can find them in vegetable oils that are on every shelf—corn oil, safflower oil, and soy bean oil. Then, of course, there are the fatty coldwater fish we have mentioned before. Don't forget nuts of all kinds and sunflower seeds. These really have lots and lots of the proper oils for you. Cross-cultural studies show that inhabitants of the countries that surround the Mediterranean, and this means on all the sides—North Africa and Europe and the Middle East—all these people seem to be protected against heart disease more than we are because they consume large quantities of monounsaturated fats in their normal diet. I'm going to get into what's called the "Mediterranean diet" a lot later, but in great detail, and see how it practically can affect us.

The monounsaturated fats seem to be able to restore something called "endothelium dependent vasodilatation." What this refers to is the thin layer of cells that line the inside of our arteries, all the way down to the smallest one. These endothelial cells react to certain molecules, especially in our foods, when they are brought into the bloodstream, by relaxing the arterial muscles. Our arteries, even our small ones, have muscles inside that can go into spasm and narrow them, and they can relax. These molecules seem to relax the arterial muscles, allowing better blood flow over long periods of time. This might prove to be the explanation, at the molecular level, of some of the cardiovascular protection we get from the monounsaturated acids—very important. It's early research, but it's nice to know we have an explanation of why that yummy avocado or guacamole is really good for us and why we should eat more.

There was a study in the *Journal of Nutritional Biochemistry* that showed that the nutritional elements in the food, such as the avocado, are markedly protective from lots and lots of diseases. Again, we need the food and not just the extract. We don't know what else was in that avocado that made it work so well. It may be a long time before we know. If you include avocado in a salad, first of all, it enhances the absorption of things like alpha-carotene, beta-carotene, and lutein—more than just the salad itself. It gets into your blood better. If you take a salsa, avocado, enhances the absorption of the lycopene and the beta-carotene. Eat the good stuff. It's going to be good for you and it'll make you happy.

Speaking of good stuff, there are some other ones that we really like. These are nuts. There's a Spanish study which was really interesting. They took groups and they gave them a daily serving of mixed nuts. They found that it improved the symptoms of metabolic syndrome—which I'm going to talk to you about later, but it's bad—obesity, high cholesterol, high blood pressure, and high blood sugar in elderly patients. What they did was they looked at 1,200 people in Spain, aged 55 to 80, who were in increased danger of getting heart disease. They studied the entire group. They divided them into separate groups. Two of them were put on the Mediterranean diet. Again, we'll talk about that later.

One of those two groups also took an additional liter of olive oil every week. That's a lot of olive oil, but it certainly could try to prove the point. The other group consumed, instead of the olive oil, an additional ounce of mixed nuts every day, a small handful of mixed nuts. Then, the control group, the third group, was put on a very nice low-fat diet and compared with the other two. In one year, there were decreases in measurable symptoms of heart disease that were 14 percent lower in the group who ate the nuts. That's a big drop. It was only 7 percent lower in the group with the extra olive oil, and just 2 percent in the control group that were eating the low-fat diets.

The omega-3 fatty acids in seeds and nuts help prevent a lot of disease—again, heart disease, and recurring heart attacks. They lower high cholesterol and triglycerides. They decrease what's called "platelet aggregation." Platelets are little particles in the blood that look like a broken plate. That's how they got their name. They immediately go to areas of inflammation or bleeding. But, in areas of inflammation, they can cause clotting. We like our platelet aggregation to be as little as possible. They reduce inflammation in the blood and they reduce blood pressure. The message really is to keep these delicious nuts and all kinds of food that you like that have the omega-3s handy. Allocate yourself a small handful every day as a snack. Don't eat a giant bowlful, which is full of a lot of fat when you get to that point. Just a little bit can make you happy—to fill you up a little bit between meals and to get all these effects.

Remember, the quality of the fat is more important than the total fat in the diet. When you can, substitute vegetable fats for animal fats. Substitute fish proteins for animal proteins. Replace whole milk with skim milk or 1 or 2 percent milk to decrease the load of saturated fats while giving you the other good things in the milk, like calcium. Eliminate solid margarine, commercially baked goods, deep fried and fast foods, to reduce the consumption of trans-fatty acids—which, ideally, you'd like to get rid of entirely. As alternatives for cooking, spreads, or baking, use oils with higher amounts of monounsaturated or polyunsaturated fatty acids—particularly the ones with the omega-3s such as olive oil and canola oil. They should basically be your cooking oils without any of the others. You can also use broth for cooking instead of oil and save the oil for your salads or for your dressings on vegetables. We'll talk a lot about that later.

We'll move on, now, in the next lecture and look at some of the foods that can be problematic for many people—especially if consumed in large quantities. We'll focus on some of the culprits for many of the diseases that medicine erroneously attributes to normal aging.

Sugar, Salt, Allergies, and Additives
Lecture 17

The consumption of added refined sugars is always terrible, and they wreak havoc in our diets. This is one area where you really do have control. You can make changes in the kinds of sugar you eat and the amount of sugar you eat. You'll receive huge health benefits from it.

This lecture looks at some foods and our responses to them that are not always optimally healthy. We'll start with sugars. As with fats, there are good sugars that are vital to our well-being, and there are bad sugars that, in overabundance, are the source of poor health. Again, as with fats, we come back to quality and quantity. The natural sugar in fruits, when eaten proportionally with other healthy foods, is quite beneficial.

A useful measure of sugar in foods is the **glycemic index**, which ranks carbohydrates based on the rate of conversion of the carbohydrate to glucose inside the body and its entrance into the bloodstream. The glycemic index is an arbitrary scale of 0 to 100, with pure glucose given a value of 100. The relevance to us is that spikes or rapid drops in blood glucose levels are unhealthy. A rapid rise in blood glucose causes an outpouring of insulin from the pancreas, which in turn can send blood glucose levels back down in a rapid overreaction. Over many years, this can lead to insulin resistance and, eventually, type 2 diabetes. Evidence seems to point to a strong correlation between high-carbohydrate diets and the development of insulin resistance.

Exercise definitely benefits long-term lowering of the blood pressure.

Some studies suggest that fructose is no better as a simple sugar than glucose is and may, in some ways, be worse. One study found that the fat gained from too much fructose has a tendency to be deposited in the organs inside the abdomen and around the belly, while glucose-generated fat tends to be stored under the skin. Research also suggests that it is dangerous to have more fat around the middle than lower in the body.

The abnormalities of blood chemistry related to the overuse of sugar are part of what's called metabolic syndrome. This is medically defined as the presence of at least three of the following factors: abdominal obesity or central obesity, high blood pressure, high triglycerides in the blood, low HDL cholesterol in the blood, and high blood glucose. It's estimated that about 25 percent of the world's adult population has metabolic syndrome. The solution is to minimize or eliminated refined sugar and maximize foods that are high in fiber and protein.

Another significant threat to our overall health is salt. The body seeks to reduce excess sodium by retaining water and filling the blood vessels too full, which elevates blood pressure. About 25 percent of all Americans have high blood pressure, and another 25 or 30 percent are considered prehypertensive. Reducing sodium intake, minimizing meat consumption, reducing alcohol, increasing fish intake, and decreasing caffeine can all help reduce blood pressure.

Food allergies are unexpected and unintended reactions that can be caused by even small amounts of a particular molecule. Common allergenic foods include dairy, eggs, nuts, seafood, tomatoes, and wheat. Preservatives and additives in food also cause problems for many people. Food sensitivities and intolerance are not related to the allergic immune-mediated response. The general advice for allergies, intolerance, and sensitivities is to read food labels carefully.

Finally, there is no evidence that detox of any kind works. Enemas, laxatives, diuretics, and transdermal detox pads have no value at all. ∎

Important Terms

food allergies: Unexpected, unintended reactions to various foods or substances in foods.

glycemic index: A numerical index that ranks carbohydrates (on a scale of 0 to 100) based on the rate of conversion of the carbohydrate to glucose inside the body and its entrance into the bloodstream.

Sugar, Salt, Allergies, and Additives
Lecture 17—Transcript

Welcome back again. We've just covered a lot of material about some really healthy foods that support optimal health.

Now let's take a look at some of the foods and some of our responses to those foods that are not always optimally healthy. We'll start with my favorite food group—sugars. I say favorite because I, as many others, have a sweet tooth. I am always challenged in finding a balance in satisfying my sweet tooth and not getting too much sugar. I grew up with enormous amounts of sugar in my diet as part of the culture of the 1940s and '50s, and unfortunately, it still is. I'm not alone. Since the 1970s, the percentage increase in sugar consumption in the United States has absolutely gone through the roof.

We humans evolved as having a natural taste for sweetness that came from our need to get as much sugar as possible in this quest to stave off starvation. Starvation was a very big threat as we evolved along the years. Sugar, when it's found in whole food, has been given a bad rap. It probably doesn't deserve that. For example, fruits, when eaten whole, with their peel and their pulp, are some of the healthiest foods in our entire nutritional world. However, refined sugars, including especially high-fructose corn syrups and some others, when added to the processed foods—especially sodas and baked goods—are an insidious part of the problem for many, many aspects of health.

As with fats, there are good sugars that are vital to our well-being, and there are bad sugars that, in overabundance, are the source of poor health. Again, as with fats, we come back to quality and to quantity. The natural sugar in fruits, when eaten proportionally with other healthy foods, are actually quite beneficial. They can add a natural sweetness to our diets, which we like. We have to keep in mind the difference between simple sugars—like sucrose, fructose, glucose—and complex carbohydrates, which I talked to you about in Lecture 12.

How do we measure sugars in foods? How do we keep track of this? Food labels only tell us the number of grams of carbohydrates and this, in turn, tells us the calories. We multiply by four; there are four calories in every gram of carbohydrates, no matter what the carbohydrate is.

If you took a packet of sugar, it has 14 grams in it. It has 4 calories per gram, so you get 56 calories in a packet of sugar. It's not very helpful because we have no idea of the amounts, for example, and the proportions in other foods that might be complex carbohydrates versus simple sugars in most foods. In the sugar packet, it's all simple sugar. But, we're going to see a lot of carbohydrates in other foods we eat, and we want to be looking for complex ones. The labels in the food, especially in the processed food boxes, don't tell us that.

A much more useful measure might be something called the "Glycemic Index." "Glycemic" means sugar in the blood. This is a numerical index that ranks carbohydrates based on the rate of conversion of the carbohydrate to glucose inside your body and entering the blood stream. They give it an arbitrary scale of 0 to 100. Pure glucose is given an arbitrary Glycemic Index of 100.

The relevance to us is that spikes and rapid increases in blood glucose levels are unhealthy, they feel horrible, and the body and many of our organs don't respond well to this. The same thing with sudden drops in these levels—they really feel awful too. Insulin is the hormone, as you know, which comes from the pancreas and reacts to blood sugar levels. It forces the sugar level out of the blood and into cells primarily in the liver where it's stored as glycogen. That's our storage of glucose precursor.

A rapid rise in blood glucose causes a huge outpouring of insulin from the pancreas, which in turn can send the blood glucose levels back down in an overreaction too rapidly—as well as causing a much more chronic condition, after many years, called "insulin resistance." In your guidebook, I have included a link to a website where you can find out the various glycemic indices of lots of different foods.

Insulin resistance is a condition where normal levels of insulin are no longer sufficient to get the normal insulin reaction from our major tissues such as fat, muscle, liver, and so on. Eventually, the pancreas can't supply enough of the body's need for insulin. Therefore, glucose levels tend to rise in the blood and eventually we end up with what's called "Type 2 diabetes," or "adult-onset diabetes."

The results of this cause a whole bunch of unpleasant, unhealthy symptoms that a diabetic has much of the time if they're not under good control. It also is accompanied by all the morbidity, such as cardiovascular heart disease, high blood pressure, strokes, and so on. Evidence seems to be pointing to a very strong correlation between high carbohydrate diets and the development of insulin resistance. Also, inactivity and obesity are contributing factors. You're going to hear me talk more and more about inactivity as opposed to the value of exercise.

Fructose and glucose—these are the two sugars you'll hear about a lot and one question continues to arise. It is whether it's healthier to take fructose as a sweetener, as added sweetener, than it is to use glucose. This is because fructose seems to be natural. It comes in fruits, and it comes in fruits that have more complex carbohydrates. They do have more complex carbohydrates. But, evidence suggests that fructose itself is no better as a simple sugar than glucose is. Some small studies now are pointing to the possibility that in some ways, fructose may actually be worse. Remember, we're getting a lot of fructose in our processed foods in the form of high-fructose corn syrup because it's very cheap and available in America.

One clinical study found that the fat gained when you have too much fructose has a tendency to be deposited in what's called the "visceral organs"—the organs inside your abdomen, and around the so-called belly, the central obesity. However, glucose-generated fat tends to be stored under the skin, where it's safer. I'm going to talk to the distribution effect when we talk about obesity. But, right now, remember that it is dangerous to have more fat around the middle, around your waist, than lower down. It's unsettled science, but it is getting to be more and more consistent in the findings. There is lots of research, lots of controversy, especially around the use of high-fructose corn syrup.

When we look at all the abnormalities related to the overuse of sugar, taken as a unit, the abnormalities of blood chemistry are part of what we call the "metabolic syndrome." I've mentioned that word before so we can define it now. The metabolic syndrome is medically defined as the presence of at least three of the following factors: abdominal obesity or central obesity, high blood pressure, high triglycerides in the blood, low HDL cholesterol in the blood, and high blood glucose. The metabolic syndrome increases a person's risk of breast cancer, cardiovascular disease, diabetes, prostate cancer, and many others. These things are unrelated, but we get them all from metabolic syndrome.

It's estimated that about 25 percent of the entire world's adults have metabolic syndrome. This causes about a three-fold increase in patients to have heart attack and strokes, and a doubling of the likelihood that they're going to die from heart attack and strokes. And they also have a five-fold increase in Type 2 diabetes. In fact, it accounts for greater morbidity and mortality throughout the world than even HIV and AIDS.

There are some general guidelines. What can we do about this? First of all, you really want to think about minimizing or even eliminating refined sugar, table sugar, soft drinks, which are loaded with sugar, and artificially sweetened fruit drinks. Carbonated soft drinks are one of the single biggest sources of calories in the American diet, especially in children and teenagers. The recent introduction of these so-called vitamin waters and health waters are especially harmful because they are generally loaded with sugar—maybe as much as 33 grams of it in a single bottle—creating more harm than the unproven good that they are promoting.

The solutions to this include maximizing foods high in fiber such as peas, beans, whole grains, and oat bran. They all have a much lower Glycemic Index, and even if you have some sugar in that meal, they'll prevent or slow down the surge of glucose in your blood stream. You can get all your carbohydrates that you would like, but you won't get the enormous blood glucose rise, and then followed by a compensatory decline in blood glucose.

Eat foods high in protein, such as rice, dairy, beans, and tofu, because they tend to have a lower Glycemic Index. Again, sugars from whole food sources and complex carbohydrates are absolutely critical to a healthy diet. The consumption of added refined sugars is always terrible, and they wreak havoc in our diets. This is one area where you really do have control. You can make changes in the kinds of sugar you eat and the amount of sugar you eat. You'll receive huge health benefits from it.

Turning to another very important potential threat to our overall health—that is salt. Salt, or what we know as sodium chloride, is really a substance that we are concerned about mostly in the sodium part of it. The chloride is not that important, it just comes along for the ride. Many people tolerate a large excess of sodium, but people with heart disease and kidney disease don't. Sodium can elevate blood pressure through several mechanisms, and one of which is you need to have a certain osmotic pressure, a certain solution level in your body. When you have a lot of sodium, the body needs to dilute it back to the proper amount. That means water retention and filling our vascular tank—our blood vessels—too full. That elevates blood pressure. Kidney responses are rather complicated, but they also tend to end up raising blood pressure.

About 25 percent of all Americans have high blood pressure, by which we mean a blood pressure over 120/80. About 25 or 30 percent, additionally, are considered prehypertensive. That means a lot of their time is spent over the normal, and a little bit of it below the normal. We have to watch them for the point where they finally become consistently hypertensive because they need treatment.

A very high percentage of African Americans and Hispanic Americans have full-blown hypertension—probably from a combination of genes and diet as well. Blood pressure increases with age for lots of us for many, many factors, but one of which is hardening of the arteries, the atherosclerosis, dietary factors in genes. Our arteries just get filled with plaques and fat, which makes them less distensible. It keeps them hard, like a rusty pipe, and building up pressure that doesn't get dissipated with the soft vessels that younger or normal people have.

High sodium diets in America happen to have become the norm. Eighty percent of dietary salt in this country—80 percent—comes from processed foods, from restaurant foods, and from fast foods because it tastes good. We like salt, and our genes tell us that salt tastes good. The recommended upper limit, for a normal diet, should probably be no more than about 2,300 mg a day. All you really need is about 1,500 mg a day.

Processed foods leave you with no choice—you have to have too much sodium. You're going to eat the food, it's going to taste good, and you're going to have an enormous amount of sodium that you're going to have to process and get rid of. Sodium reduction also decreases blood pressure in hypertensive people and borderline hypertensive people, so just decreasing that amount can help them without any medication.

The first line of attack in treating people who are hypertensive is to just decrease the sodium intake. Decreases which have been shown to go from 4,000 mg—which is not unusual in this country—down to 2,000 mg—which I consider high, but it's about average—results in a small change. This is about two or three millimeters of mercury, of pressure measurement. This is for the short term. It's not a very big change. People would say, why bother? However, over the long term, a one percent change, can reduce blood pressure by as much as 10 millimeters of mercury, which starts to get substantial. That brings the risk down and is worth achieving.

Remember that other than having vessels that are hardened and narrowed, there are other problems with high blood pressure itself. It forces the heart to expend a lot more energy on every single stroke, and it pumps just to get the blood around the body against this head of pressure. It also creates physical exertion and stress on lots of other organs which don't like hypertension. The kidney is one that can be harmed by high blood pressure. It expedites the whole aging process. Again, the results of high blood pressure, the heart disease, the stroke, and the kidney all tend to make life worse, less healthy, and often shorter.

While we're on the topic of this, there are some things that you can do to help reduce blood pressure. For example, a vegetarian diet can often help, or at least minimizing meat consumption. Reducing alcohol—there's a very, very strong relationship between alcohol and high blood pressure. Of course, increasing the fish intake we talked about. Decreasing caffeine—small amounts of caffeine, a cup or two of coffee a day, a little bit of tea probably may even be beneficial, but it certainly doesn't hurt. But, when you get up there—five, six, seven, cups of coffee—it's going to raise your blood pressure over long periods of time. That's not good. Exercise definitely benefits long-term lowering of the blood pressure. You're going to hear more and more as we progress about how exercise kind of trumps almost everything else in its benefits. Weight loss itself, just reducing the weight, will bring down the blood pressure.

There is no proof that lowering salt intake in a normal individual will reduce their blood pressure, decrease heart disease, or help them with longevity. People with normal blood pressure just seem to do okay with how they handle sodium. Small changes in normal blood pressure—let's say from going from 115/75 to 110/70—those small changes have not been shown to make any difference in health outcomes, so you really can ignore them.

The tip of the day about sodium is, again, not only moderation, but if you really like that taste—and who doesn't like the taste of salt, it makes things taste good—you need to cut down your sodium. You want to keep the better taste, and you're finding your food too bland. What you can do is keep your sodium on top of the food so that the salt gets to your tongue first. If you take mashed potatoes and you mix in your allowance of sodium, it's going to get diluted. You won't taste it as much, so you'll want to use more; you won't feel good about it. If you take your potatoes and put a little bit of sodium right on top, take a spoonful of that, or a forkful, and you'll taste it right away. It's going to hit the tongue first and less sodium will go a long way.

We've explored the issues of sugar and salt and the havoc they wreak on our health. I want to point you to a new book called *The End of Overeating* by Dr. David Kessler. It's in our bibliography, and I highly recommend that you read the whole thing. He's explained how those two combined—sugar and salt—with the addition of fat, have created a huge nutritional demon. There is a craving for food that Kessler explains. Kessler, by the way, is a Harvard-trained doctor. He is a lawyer. He is a medical school dean, and he was the former commissioner of the Food and Drug Administration. He knows what he's talking about. There's a lot of science in his books.

Foods, he has found, that are high in sugar, salt, and fat can actually alter our brain chemistry and promote overeating. The salt, fat, sugar combinations found, again, in fast foods, processed foods, and restaurant food stimulate the brain to crave still more. Do you remember the old potato chips ad that said, "Betcha can't eat just one"? They were right. Who can eat one? It's fat, it's sugar, and it's salty. It's delicious. The brain just loves it. Processed foods—whether they are intentionally loaded with this stuff or it just happens to be in there—they are designed to make you want more.

Let's move on now, and we'll talk about other food sources that cause different reactions in different people. There's a lot of discussion these days about different types of food allergies, food sensitivities, and food intolerance. I'll talk to you now about how they differ and how they might affect us.

First are food allergies. These are what we call in medicine "idiosyncratic reactions," meaning unexpected, unintended reactions. Even small amounts of a particular molecule can cause these. They're often foreign species proteins, like eggs, that come from a chicken instead of a human, or shellfish. They're mediated by definition by our immune system through something called "immunoglobulin E" or "IgE" antibodies. We can measure these. They can be mild. They can be something as simple, for example, as a runny nose or some phlegm. But, they can also be very fast in onset and very severe and fatal within minutes in the most severe reactions. Some milder symptoms that are unpleasant, but not fatal, can include vomiting, diarrhea, bloody stools, itching, hives, wheezing when you try to breathe—all kinds of reactions can occur in different people to different extents.

The reactions are mediated often by the release of a substance called "histamine," which is why we take antihistamines. They cause most of the symptoms of this immune overreaction, like the wheezing, respiratory distress, and anaphylactic shock. That's a term referring to a kind of shock that rapidly occurs, meaning a blood pressure lowering, and often death in cases of severe allergy. The responses can be immediate or they can be delayed. They can be severe; they can be mild. Anaphylactic shock can occur in minutes. A patient can be dead in two minutes.

The main diagnosis of food allergy is usually by history—careful history, because it's very difficult to separate the ingredients—skin testing, and even blood testing for these IgE antibodies. Some of the most common ones that top the list of allergenic foods include dairy, eggs, nuts—very common—seafood, wheat, and cow's milk—one of the most common. How often have you taken ice cream or milk and find that all of a sudden you're getting a little bit of phlegm, not paying attention? It's not severe. It's usually an allergic response to a protein that came out of a cow that you're not familiar with or that your body recognizes as a foreign protein. Tomatoes are very allergenic. We've all heard stories about the tragedies from peanuts. Peanuts can be fatal with exposure to a few molecules of it if you're allergic. If you're not allergic, it doesn't make any difference. They all contain some foreign protein, so they're fair game for the immune system to recognize as foreign.

Food sensitivities and intolerance are kind of hard to differentiate and define differently. I like to look at them together. They are not related to the immune system response. They're quite different. People say allergy when it may be sensitivity or intolerance. About 30 percent of our population experience some episodes of food sensitivity some of the time. They're very, very vague. They're very difficult to pinpoint.

They are more likely to be a toxic reaction to the food rather than an allergic immune mediated response. They're generally similar symptoms to the allergies, but often more vague like persistent fatigue, gas and bloating, nervousness, anxiety, and mild headaches. They are very difficult to diagnose because there's a time lag. They usually don't occur immediately. You can eat the food now and get signs and symptoms later or the next day. There's a lot of poor recall about what you might have eaten in your meals, and most meals contain several elements. Which one was it?

It's often a diagnosis of exclusion—what we call elimination diet. You start removing one thing from your diet at a time until you see that you no longer get the symptoms. This can take a long time. It took me 30 years to figure out that I was very, very sensitive to artificial food dyes. Then, you start putting things back in your diet. You try your sensitive food again, and you see if it causes you symptoms. There are many, many different reactions, failure to digest certain substances—very common—most commonly, things like lactose, gluten, and preservatives.

The general advice on allergies, intolerance, and sensitivities—what should you do if you think you have this or you do have it? Read your labels carefully. Most of the stuff that you might have a problem with is on those labels. Avoid processed foods as much as you possibly can because you don't really know what's in there. Not everything in there is on the label. This is because, for example, if it's not organic, then you're going to have chemicals, pesticides, some toxins that may have gotten on to the food, but which haven't been defined by the manufacturer. Sticking to fresh, organic produce is going to eliminate some of that problem.

The role of preservatives and additives is a really big, emerging science today. One more of my reasons for the emphasis on the inclusion of real food and the exclusion of processed and fake food is the presence of these additives in all of them. They include: benzoates, which are in thousands of foods; sulfites, which are in wine; butylated hydroxytoluene, which is a preservative; flavoring agencies and dyes are all problems for a lot of people.

There's a Center for Science in the Public Interest which is in your website list in our bibliography. They reviewed the research showing commonly used food dyes and petrochemicals like Yellow Dye 5—I'm sure you've seen that—Red Dye 40, and lots of others. They have now been seriously linked, in children, to attention deficit hyperactivity disorders, hyperactivity itself, impulsivity, and learning difficulties. The FDA has been petitioned along with the food industry to ban these dyes. There has already been a recommendation by some of the countries in Europe to phase them out completely.

Finally, there's the issue of age. Allergies are more common in infants than in adults. Six to eight percent of infants and children experience some food allergies, but they often outgrow it. Children and younger people are also much more sensitive to dose because these preservatives, synthetic chemicals, and sugar and salt itself, tends to be more of a relative dose in their smaller bodies. They are very much more vulnerable. Bad habits that they develop in eating are much harder to change. Their bodies are forming and changing and the imbalances have a long-term consequence for them.

Sensitivities are more prevalent in the adults. Aging is often accompanied by a less effective digestive tract. Their digestive enzymes are on the wane and decline, and GI function diminishes some. Lactose intolerance, which just means you can't break down milk sugar and causes a lot of symptoms, is much more common over the age of 40. It's just a failure, a general decline in the GI tract.

One final topic, which I can't leave you without talking about, is the lucrative medical scams about detox. There is no evidence that detox of any kind actually works. They are of no value, and they are potentially harmful. Don't do anything with enemas, laxatives, diuretics, or these transdermal detox pads. They have no value at all. They just take your money, and they will lead you to great disappointment. Especially colon cleansing and coffee enemas; they're unnecessary. They have no benefit. Your own colon does a magnificent job, if unromantic, at cleaning your insides. No help is needed and there are lots of risks.

There are a wide variety of foods which may evoke unpleasant and unhealthy responses in you and different people and at different levels. Sulfites in wines, nitrates and nitrites in meat wreak havoc with many of us. Others can be allergic to shellfish, mushrooms, fruits, and vegetables that have substances added. Track these down if you can, and get rid of them.

In the next lecture, we'll move on to ways in which our body responds to foods in general and how absorption varies from one person to another, often in very different ways, even in the same family.

The Physiology of Weight Management
Lecture 18

There is no doubt in my mind that physical inactivity is dangerous across the majority of health and risk factors. Just as important, activity and exercise are beneficial across all risk and health factors. Moderate levels of obesity are not nearly as detrimental when compared to inactivity.

Obesity is one of the fastest growing disease epidemics in our country. The CDC estimates that about 66 percent of Americans fall into the overweight category, and 33 percent are considered severely obese. Obesity is the third leading preventable cause of death in the United States, behind smoking and high blood pressure.

Will power is not the answer to weight control. Genes help establish the body structure, and the brain and body physiology fight to defend that structure. The body's drive toward stable weight maintenance is very efficient, which is why dieting alone rarely succeeds. The BMI is the most standardized measure of weight. It's calculated by multiplying weight in pounds by 703, then dividing by height in inches squared.

Humans have evolved hundreds of genes to stave off starvation. When you go on a diet, the body responds first by lowering its metabolic rate to try to stop weight loss. This is why dieters generally experience a plateau after losing a few pounds. The metabolism has been processing 2,000 calories a day, but if you cut out 500, the body will reset its own metabolic level down to 1,500. Hunger signals will also increase.

Interestingly, how your body burns calories can be influenced by the geographical origins of your ancestors. The genes of people who have ancestors from cold environments have adapted so that their bodies use fewer calories to make more heat. Australian Aboriginal cultures had to evolve using calories from the very few edible fats and proteins in their environment. The good news is that it's not impossible to fight nature in this regard.

Excess weight distribution by body shape is critical and is also highly determined by genes. People with **apple-shaped bodies** (weight concentrated around the waist) are at increased risk for diabetes, heart disease, high blood pressure, and stroke. An expanded waist size reflects total and intra-abdominal fat, which for some reason is metabolically more active. It can move to other parts of the body, such as the arteries.

A number of studies suggest you don't have to be thin to be healthy. Even people who are as much as 20 pounds over normal weight can be fit and healthy, and it may be better to accept some degree of overweight than to subject yourself to yo-yo dieting.

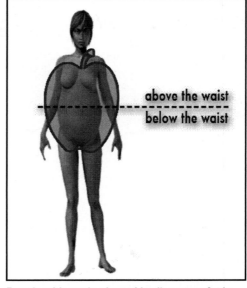

People with apple-shaped bodies store fat in their midsections, above and below the navel.

Spot reducing, fad diets, and special weight-loss suits don't work. The key is to gradually make permanent, sustainable lifestyle changes. Add more fruits and vegetables to your diet, supplemented with nuts and other healthy snacks. Eat until you are no longer hungry rather than until you're full, be aware of portion sizes, and eat slowly. Eat a substantial breakfast, a slightly lighter lunch, and an even lighter dinner. Movement is an absolute must to counterbalance your body's efforts to thwart weight loss.

For morbidly obese people, bariatric surgery may be necessary. This involves either stapling the upper portion of the stomach, creating a very small pouch for food, or bypassing much of the small intestine where food absorption takes place. Both these procedures have some good results for people who are desperately at risk, but they also carry their own dangers. ■

apple-shaped body: A body shape with more weight around the waist than around the hips.

Questions to Consider

1. Name five health-threatening conditions associated with obesity.

2. Explain why a low-calorie diet may work for weight loss in the short term but not in the long term.

The Physiology of Weight Management
Lecture 18—Transcript

Welcome back. We've talked about the physiology of how our bodies respond to different foods and the importance of the quality and the quantity. Today we're going to look at one of the fastest growing disease epidemics in the country—the issue of obesity and weight management in general.

Obesity especially is a very painful subject for many people, not only physiologically, but also socially, emotionally, and financially. The cost to our health system is enormous. There's a lot of important terminology that we're going to have to try to deal with. Let's acknowledge that some of the terms are misunderstood. For example, the idea of being overweight or obese, or being thin or fit—all of these have different meanings to different people. They're vague. We have to see what we're really talking about before we move into any kind of a scientific discussion.

Weight in pounds or kilograms does not give us a solid definition. It needs to be correlated with height as well and with the composition of the weight. With regards to obesity, I'll try to talk about two different groups in general rather than getting down into very fine divisions. We want to talk about, on the one hand, mild to moderate weight—which can include most of us who are trying to lose some weight—and severe obesity, which is in a growing number of individuals, but still a minority.

The facts are that most Americans gain about an average of more than one to one-and-a-half pounds every year between the ages of 20 and 40. This adds up to about 30 pounds of excess weight by the time they reach 40 to 50. An increase in calorie intake of only 15 calories a day, in a diet that may be 2,000 calories, could account for that weight gain. That's really one degree of change in a very bad way.

The CDC estimates that about 66 percent of Americans are going to fall into the overweight category; 33 percent can be considered severely obese. That's a very big number. Fewer fall into the very far end of the extreme called morbid obesity—and I'll define that for you later—and 17 percent of our children are obese, and that percentage is rising all the time. Obesity is the third leading preventable cause of death in the United States behind smoking and high blood pressure. Of course, with high blood pressure, it tends to be related.

Will power is not the answer to weight control. Genes help establish the body structure, and the brain and body physiology fight to defend that structure. The body's drive towards stable weight maintenance is very, very efficient. Dieting alone rarely succeeds. The body can bypass the lower caloric intake. Relapse rates for obesity tend to be very high. The most successful programs avoid the thousands of fad diets. In my last visit to a big chain bookstore, I counted over 300 diet books. Only the Bible outsells diet books.

Here's another rule that I learned long ago when I was a resident. I was about to do an operation for a hiatal hernia, which is a disease where the stomach protrudes up into the chest. There were four operations named after the inventors—the Allison, the Hill, the Belsey, and the Nissen. I went to my professor and said, "Which one should we do?" He said, "It doesn't matter." What this tells you is that, when you have four operations for one disease, if one of those operations was actually any better, everyone would be doing it.

It's the same with diet. If one diet worked, we wouldn't have 300 diet books. If we measure the body in its mass index, this is the most standardized measure of weight. It's the one measure that does take height into consideration, and there are calculators you can go to on the Internet to make it very easy, just plugging in your numbers. Basically, your body mass index is your weight in pounds, times 703, divided by your height in inches squared. Height is very important because we're squaring that value.

If you weigh 160 pounds and you're 5-foot-10 or 70 inches, your BMI is 160 times 703 divided by 4,900, or 22.9—which is normal. If you look at the table in the guidebook, this puts you into the normal category. If you look below and above that, you'll see what numbers change your body mass index. Remember, we square the height. The height is important, and it doesn't change. Therefore, it takes a lot of change in your weight to change where you fall on that table.

This scale has other variations, if you see it other places, as to the categories of obese or severely obese. But, we'll use this one for consistency. The BMI is admittedly not the perfect measure of obesity, but it's a guide. It doesn't measure, for example, the percent of body fat which is another good indicator of obesity. It may not apply in special situations—for example, in athletes, who have a very large amount of muscle but who might still have a higher BMI than normal because their weight is higher, but it's not fat.

When necessary, we can look to other measurements. For now, I'm going to use the BMI as a base of comparison. There's a really important physiology fact that you want to keep in mind in this search. Your body wants to maintain its weight. We evolved hundreds and hundreds of genes just to stave off starvation because starvation was by far the greatest risk, more than almost anything else in evolution. Certainly, up to a certain point, obesity wasn't a risk at all. It's a greater risk, in fact, than almost all the other risks put together. When we go on extreme diets, or any diet to lose weight, the body will respond first and immediately by lowering its metabolic rate to try to stop the loss. This is like turning down the thermostat so you use less fuel to heat your room. It is just perceived as too great a threat by our genes.

When you go on a diet, the first thing that happens generally is you lose a lot of water. You think you've lost weight. Then, the caloric effect kicks in. If you normally eat 2,000 calories in a day, and you decide to knock off 500 of those, that'll work for a while. You'll lose a few pounds very early on, and then suddenly we all notice we level off because the body resets the thermostat. It takes its own metabolic level down to 1,500. You're now going to have to move down another few hundred calories, which gets much harder to do, in order to continue to lose weight.

This is why crash diets and extreme diets only succeed for a very short period of time, and why so many people regress back to their other weight. The body doesn't want you to do this. When it senses starvation, it swings into a high-gear survival mode. It does everything it can do to prevent further weight loss. All its mechanisms are aimed at defending your weight. It wants to keep defeating your weight loss program. Reductions in metabolic rate are one way, and it increases all your hunger signals. You will be hungry all the time. Over the past couple of decades, we've learned that the body strives to maintain the weight by a whole bunch of redundant controls. Intervening in any one of those triggers compensatory reaction by the body to offset whatever challenge you're giving it.

The body's obesity has a big impact on function and structure. Because of the burden of the extra weight on other parts of the body, the additional weight—as well as the additional blood flow circulating to the new fat in the body and in other systems—and bearing weight on your joints creates a lot of additional risks. The organs of your body and the muscles all have to work harder. Your knees, your hips have to support the weight, and they take a lot more trauma.

The question comes up about genes versus environment in the whole problem of obesity. It turns out, unfortunately, that genetics are critically important. How your body burns calories can be influenced by the geography of origin of your long-dead ancestors. The mitochondrial DNA is maternally inherited, and it differs by geography. The genes of those, for example, who have ancestors who came from cold, arctic environments have adapted so that their bodies use fewer calories to make more heat. Indigenous populations such as Australian Aboriginal cultures had to evolve using calories from the very few edible fats and proteins in their environment, which was very, very sparse. They had to be very efficient just to survive.

There was a study very recently that looked at Aboriginal experiences in Australia. There were subjects who had moved to cities and had developed Type 2 diabetes. They were insulin resistant, they had metabolic syndrome, and they volunteered to go back to their Aboriginal homelands. They lived as their Aboriginal partners did, and they ate only indigenous foods. In seven weeks, there was a marked improvement in all the parameters that you could measure in this metabolic syndrome.

Other studies on identical twins who were raised apart by other families strongly suggest that there's a very powerful influence from the genes. Twins who were born to at least one obese family member and raised in a family of very thin individuals almost always became obese. There was an even stronger correlation when both parents of the original biologic side were obese.

But, we also know that how people live accounts for more than half of the difference in the quality and the longevity of life until they die—the old nurture and environment aspect that can help defeat some of the natural propensities of the genes. It may be difficult to fight nature, but it's not impossible. Good habits started very early in life are likely to have the greatest health benefits. The greatest lifelong gift you can give your kids and your grandkids is the establishment of healthy habits while they're very young.

Let's move on and talk a little bit about body shape. I think most of us are really very focused on our body shape. Excess weight distribution by body shape happens to be absolutely critical. It's something many people always thought about. They said well, I always gain my weight here or I gain my weight there or I can't lose it here—and they happen to be right. Specific distribution of fat in the body is very highly determined by the genes.

You all suspected this, and you were right. It's very easily seen, and very easily measured. If you measure the circumference of the waist versus the circumference of your hips, if excess weight is concentrated around your waist, above your hips—which makes you a little top heavy—then, they call this "apple shaped." Technically, we call it "central obesity." If the excess weight, on the other hand, is concentrated lower, down around the hips and the thighs—making you bottom heavy—then the body is what they call "pear shaped." The difference between apple and pear shape is significant.

Apple-shaped bodies are far more dangerous and are at increased risk for diabetes, heart disease, high blood pressure, and stroke. There is now no question about that. The pear-shaped bodies have more difficulty dieting and exercising to alter the shape, but they don't have that increased risk. An individual's expanded waist size reflects total as well as intra-abdominal fat—fat that's inside your abdomen surrounding your internal, or what we call "visceral," organs. That fat, for some reason, is metabolically more active. It can move around to other parts of the body that may be dangerous to your health, like your arteries. The risks increase many fold in men whose waists, in general, measure more than 40 inches around, and in women who measure more than 35 inches around. It's a really easy measure to do. You can get a lot of information and this is something you need to focus on.

Which would you rather be? Would you rather be thin or would you rather be fit? Which is more important? There are a number of studies. They're a little confusing, but I think we can draw some conclusions. A number of the studies suggest you don't have to be thin to be healthy. It's pretty well accepted now that people with even as much as 20 pounds or more over what's considered normal weight can be very fit, and they can be healthy. It may be better to stay fit and accept some degree of being overweight than to beat yourself up with yo-yo dieting and a lot of guilt just to get off those last few pounds.

Some people spend their lives dieting, losing and gaining hundreds of pounds of weight. They suffer significant mental and emotional stress that's probably not good for them mentally, physiologically, or psychologically. There was a study of 900 women with heart problems. That's a big group. The women who were overweight but fit had a lower risk of all those things we keep talking about—arterial blockages, heart attacks, strokes, and other heart problems—when measured against those in the groups who were at a normal weight but unfit.

There are a lot of contradictory studies. You could really find almost anything you want to backup your argument in this. The JAMA, the *Journal of the American Medical Association*, showed that fitness and weight were significant independently of each other in both men and women. In comparing to those who were overweight but fit, those who were normal weight and unfit had a lower health risk than the other group. In another study, disease risk was lowest in people who had normal, healthy weight and were in good physical shape—no surprises there.

Then, in the nurses study, which we'll talk a lot more about later—this was a large, long-term study—it showed that physical activity decreased the rate of death for nurses of all weights. Therefore, being fit was important. Being a little overweight, when combined with doing more regular exercise, is probably a good thing. My own conclusions and my personal bias, as you'll learn in the next section on exercise, is to go for more exercise. There is no doubt in my mind that physical inactivity is dangerous across the majority of health and risk factors. Just as important, activity and exercise are beneficial across all risk and health factors. Moderate levels of obesity are not nearly as detrimental when compared to inactivity.

It is probably much more harmful to become obsessed with a number on a scale, a BMI index number, or the percentage of your body fat, than to allow yourself a little leeway in your weight and keep on moving your bodies in beneficial ways and pleasurable activities. Up to a point, the more movement the better. We'll talk much more about this when we get to exercise.

What works and what doesn't work in general? The big myth, one of the really big myths, is about spot reducing. Exercises that can take the fat off your thighs or your upper arms or your abdomen—they don't work. There is no way to spot reduce any part of the body. The body decides where the fat goes, and exercising the muscles underneath there will not do it for you. There are devices that try to jiggle the weight off your arms or contract them off with electrical stimulation. They don't work either. The rubber suit myth—that's really irrational. People dress up in rubber tops and rubber pants. They go out, and they fill their suits with sweat. Of course they lose weight, but it's all water and salt. It's totally irrational. It brings you right back to the normal weight within a few grams as soon as you rehydrate. It does no good.

There's a very rough guide to the lifestyle choices of the fit, and I think we can follow some of those choices. First of all, we want to not diet in the conventional meaning. You don't want to change your eating habits every time your weight changes. Better than this is to develop a lifelong habit—which I will cover in the next lecture—making small, permanent lifestyle changes one degree at a time that you can gradually incorporate and you can sustain. Make sensible choices in what you eat rather than the quick fix, fad diets. Remember, because there are so many diets, it really means they don't work.

You want to add more fruits and veggies, to supplement them with nuts and other healthy snacks, and have more fiber. It fills you up. It'll get rid of a lot of extra hunger. Drink lots more water. It's good for you. It'll also take away some hunger. You want to provide more food volume in your stomach for the number of calories you're getting. Remember the satiety index—how foods swell up and make you feel full, also how they get into the bloodstream and signal that you should be full. This is a measure of how full certain foods make you. You can look this up and see what might help you. It'll change the way you eat.

You also want to get into a habit that little children have. I think you've all noticed this—it's to eat until you are no longer hungry. Don't eat until you're full. This is what most of us do. We eat. We continue to eat, and then we're full and uncomfortable. If you watch the kids, they often leave food on their plate because they've satisfied their hunger.

You don't want deprivation to be part of this way of eating. You want to go for moderation, and one of them is portion control. Many of our restaurants just pile the food on the plate. Plates actually have gotten bigger over time. One of the things you can do is, if you eat with a partner, split the entrees. Maybe you both have a salad. Split the entrees, which is certainly going to be cheaper. You usually find you've had enough to eat. No deprivation, give yourself realistic goals.

You also want to remember that it helps if you eat slowly. It actually takes as long as about 20 minutes before the brain signals us that we should be feeling full—in other words, that we should stop eating. That's a delay we're not mostly cognizant of. If you eat really fast, you can overfill your stomach and bypass all those signals before your brain has a chance to react. Slow eating allows that signal to get us there before we overeat. There is a whole slow food movement which speaks to the issue of eating slowly in the proper environment. We're going to talk to that later when we get into lifestyles.

It's critical to find ways on how to slow down and find pleasure in the food. That is part of some of the longest-lived cultures that we've already looked at. We'll talk about them again. Those cultures do have a pattern of eating together, eating slowly, and eating in smaller amounts. It also helps to keep temptations out of the house, and then have a lot of healthy alternatives very conveniently placed—a glassful of carrots in the refrigerator, a bunch of blueberries, a plate of dried nuts.

Portion control, getting back to that, is absolutely critical. It's very, very sustainable and here's the reason. It's the story of the incredible shrinking stomach. I've had the experience—and most of you probably have not—of operating on someone who has just eaten a big meal, in an emergency. You can get a stomach, which is normally about that big—not very big—that can be to here, absolutely hanging down almost in their pelvis. The stomach is very stretchable. When the stomach stretches, it signals the brain to stop eating. But, now, if you're constantly eating large meals, that becomes the norm and it takes more stretching to get the signal. If you have a stomach that's used to small portions that comes from portion control or eating small meals during the day, the stomach tends to get much smaller over a long time. Then, a little bit of stretching will make you feel full. That's going to go a long way to reducing the number of calories.

Also, be aware of some of the emotional eating traps—like depression, anger, disappointment. Be aware that these are very common triggers for overeating. Comfort foods, also, from our childhood, tend to be very, very high in fats and calories. I can still smell and taste grilled cheese sandwiches with bacon on them and things that my mother gave me when I was hungry that she knew I liked. It's very easy to go back to those when you're under some stress.

The other thing is eating a substantial breakfast. This is now very, very well studied. You want a breakfast with a good satiety index because it will set you up for the rest of the day. You want to have that breakfast very well balanced. You want to have carbohydrates that get into your system fairly quickly to get you feeling good about your fullness. You want some proteins that take a little longer, and then you want some fats that stay with you.

Then, you should look to a slightly lighter lunch. Finally, at the end of the day, it should be the lightest meal of all, your dinner. The cultures with excellent longevity and health records tend to have their biggest meals around lunch or earlier. Don't skip meals; this is really a bad idea. More than about four to six hours without food is going to decrease your metabolism to compensate, so you're not going to burn many calories. You'll also get hungry. Then, you're going to eat more.

Movement is really the absolute must to counterbalance what your body is doing to thwart your weight loss. You have to be able to move more and exercise more to keep the body burning those calories. That's more than just a stroll after dinner. You're going to need to get out there and do some real physical activity.

Obesity and extreme overweight can be socially contagious. Having obese friends has now been shown to influence the way you eat toward obesity. This doesn't mean you need to leave your friends. You just need to be aware of this influence, and maybe also expand your social circle. But, be aware. As you may recall, a large and supportive community is very much part of the foundations of healthy aging. You can incorporate this whole idea of thinness into your community.

A quick word about morbid obesity—these are people who are either twice the normal weight, 100 pounds overweight, or have a BMI of more than 40. They have an extreme risk for both morbidity and mortality. They often require surgical intervention because it doesn't usually work, when you're up there at 350 pounds, to get down to any kind of a healthy weight. Before resorting to surgery, most of these people undergo medical intervention, psychological and psychiatric interventions too, but they often fail.

There are some surgical options for the treatment. I'll just mention them very quickly. This is called "bariatric surgery." It is not cosmetic surgery. It is treatment of a condition that has life-threatening consequences. There are two kinds. First, what is called "restrictive procedures of the stomach" in which you make the patient unable and not desiring to eat more than very small amounts at one time before they're uncomfortably full. I'm talking about two to three ounces, which is about that much food. What we do with those patients is we operate on them. We can either staple the upper portion of their stomach near the esophagus—making a very small pouch and a very small passage for the food to empty—or we can put different kinds of synthetic bands around it which also make a small pouch with a small opening. They eat just a little bit and then the stretching of that part of their tiny, tiny stomach pouch makes them feel full. Most of these people have been eating a lot of food for a long time. They don't really like this, but it helps and it works for them.

The other ones are bypass operations in which you bypass the 28 or 30 feet of your small intestine where all your food absorption takes place. You hook the patient back up so they only have a few feet of intestine left. Not enough can be absorbed to maintain their weight, and in fact, they lose rather rapidly. Most patients like this operation because they can continue to eat as much as they want. The only problem with it is that it's very dangerous. The nutritional aspects are very difficult to manage. Both these procedures have some very, very good results for people who are desperately at risk. They have a lot of risks too.

In summary, we're going to talk about, again, and continue to talk about, moderation, moderation, moderation in our eating. It does not include deprivation or starvation. I'm going to continue to talk about getting you to move your body often, and to periodically move it intensely. We'll talk about this in the lectures ahead, and we won't forget Goldilocks. We have to have a diet we like to eat, that pleases us. We want to enjoy the journey and find the pleasure in slowing down and eating whole foods.

We have one more lecture on nutrition in which I'll compare nutritional plans and a few diets. I'll highlight those most consistent with overall success in maintaining our diet and our well-being.

This page has been intentionally left blank.

Supplemental Material

Table 1. Body mass index

Category	BMI
Underweight	<18.5
Normal	18.5–24.9
Overweight	25–26.9
Obese	27–29.9
Moderately obese	30–34.9
Severely obese	35–39.9
Morbidly obese	>40

Note: To calculate your body mass index (BMI), multiply your weight in pounds by 703, then divide by your height in inches squared. For example, if you are 5 feet 6 inches tall and weigh 150 pounds, your BMI is calculated as follows:

$$150 \times 703 = 105,450$$
$$66^2 = 4,356$$
$$105,450 \div 4,356 = 24.2$$

Thus your weight is considered normal and healthy for your height.

Table 2. Major vitamins at a glance

Vitamin	Function	Sources and stability
Retinol (vitamin A and provitamin A)	Produces vision pigment; promotes resistance to infection and growth of healthy epithelial cells.	Fish; liver; dark orange, yellow, and red fruits and vegetables; dark green leafy fruits and vegetables. Heat stable. Destroyed by exposure to light and the type of packaging material.
Ascorbic acid/ L-ascorbic acid (vitamin C)	Maintains iron in its reduced state to preserve activity of at the catalytic site.	Fruits and vegetables, especially oranges, grapefruit, papaya, and strawberries. Destroyed by light, heat, air, iron, or copper.
Cholecalciferol (vitamin D_3)/ ergocalciferol (vitamin D_2)	Facilitates calcium absorption from the intestine and maintenance of phosphorus levels in blood. As antioxidants, prevent oxidation of unsaturated fatty acids and maintain the integrity of cell membranes.	Fatty fish, egg, liver, and fish liver oils. Available mostly in artificially fortified products, such as milk, yogurt, breakfast cereals, and breads. Very stable, but pure cholecalciferol samples are destroyed by high temperatures and humidity. Most stable form is obtained by encapsulating vitamin D_3 within a protective matrix.
Tocopherol (vitamin E)	Maintains the integrity of cell membranes.	Vegetable oils, leafy green vegetables, and whole grains (wheat germ). Destroyed by heat, light, and oxygen.
Quinones (vitamins K_1 and K_2)	Formation of several blood clotting factors in the liver. Synthesized by bacteria in the large intestine.	Green leafy vegetables and some fruits, dairy products, meat, and eggs. Moderately stable to heat and reducing agents. Destroyed by acid, alkali, light, and oxidizing agents. Best derived from food sources only.

Dietary reference intake	Disorders related to deficiency	Disorders related to toxicity
Men: 900 mcg Women: 700 mcg Upper adult limit: 2,000 mcg	Alcoholism (by precipitating zinc deficiency), celiac disease, fat malabsorption disorders, and respiratory disease.	Cheilitis (dry lips); nasal, eye, and skin mucosa dryness; hair loss, nail fragility, bone pain, gingivitis, hepatomegaly, and ascites.
Men: 90 mg Women: 75 mg Upper adult limit: 1,925 mcg (77,000 IU)	Scurvy (weakened connective tissue, lesions/impaired wound healing, poorly formed collagen).	Nausea and diarrhea (rare).
Adults, 51–70 yr: 10 mcg (400 IU) Adults >70 yr: 15 mcg Upper adult limit: 2,000 IU	Rickets, depression, abnormal functioning and premature aging.	Excess or deficiency can cause abnormal functioning and premature aging.
Adults: 15 mg Upper adult limit: 1,000 mg	Sterility, cystic fibrosis.	No known toxicity.
Men: 120 mcg Women: 90 mcg Upper adult limit: N/A	Bleeding disorders, increased risk of spontaneous hemorrhage.	Thrombogenesis, hemolysis, and increased risk of jaundice (rare).

Table 3. B vitamin information at a glance

B vitamin	Function	Sources and stability
Thiamin (B1)	Breaks down carbohydrate..	Fortified cereals, pork, and navy beans. Destroyed by heat and baking soda.
Riboflavin (B2)	Supports energy metabolism.	Liver, fortified cereals, milk, and yogurt. Destroyed by UV light.
Niacin (B3)	Supports energy metabolism.	Meat, poultry, nuts, peanuts, and cereals.
Pantothenic acid (B5)	Synthesizes coenzymes important for fatty acid energy metabolism.	Beef, poultry, potatoes, and vegetables.
Pyridoxine (B6)	Amino acid metabolism.	Liver, fish, poultry, fruits, and whole grains. Destroyed by heat.
Biotin (B7)	Fatty acid synthesis and metabolism, gluconeogenesis, and amino acid metabolism.	Liver, nuts, and eggs.
Folate (B9)	Metabolism of amino acids and synthesis of DNA; cell division and development of neural tube in fetuses.	Fortified cereal, spinach, broccoli, black and pinto beans, orange juice, and potatoes. Extremely vulnerable to heat.
Cyanocobalamin (B12)	Folate absorption; synthesis of myelin.	Liver, meat, eggs, and milk.

Dietary reference intake	Disorders related to deficiency	Disorders related to toxicity
Male, 19–70 yr: 1.2 mg Female, 19–70 yr: 1.1 mg	Beriberi; "pins and needles" sensation.	No known toxicity.
Male, 19–70 yr: 1.3 mg Female, 19–70 yr: 1.1 mg	Mouth sores and inflammation.	No known toxicity.
Male, 19–70 yr: 16 mg Female, 19–70 yr: 14 mg Upper limit, adult: 35 mg	Pellegra.	Flushing and redness.
5 mg	Rare.	No known toxicity.
Adult, 19–50 yr: 1.3 mg Male, 50–70 yr: 1.7 mg Female, 50–70 yr: 1.5 mg Upper limit, adult: 100 mg	Microcytic hypochromic anemia.	Weakness; numbness.
Adult, 19–50 yr: 30 mg	Rare.	No known toxicity.
Adult: 400 mcg Upper limit, adult: 1000 mcg	Neural tube defects in fetuses; macrocytic anemia.	No known toxicity but can mask a B12 deficiency.
Adult: 2.4 mcg	Pernicious and macrocytic anemias.	No known toxicity.

Source: Data from Northwestern University, "Nutrition Fact Sheets."
Note: yr = year; mg = milligram; mcg = microgram.

Glossary

abdominoplasty: Surgical removal of excess skin and fat to flatten out the abdomen.

absolute risk: The actual numerical chance or probability discovered during a study, presented without context, using numbers or percentages. For example, if a study of two drug treatments shows that a risk of death from using one drug is 1 out of 7,000 and the risk of death from using the second drug is 2 out of 7,000, then the difference in absolute risk is very small (a rise of only 1 death in 7,000 participants). In contrast, the **relative risk** for using the second drug (an increase from 1 to 2) shows a 100 percent increase.

acetylcholine: A neurotransmitter that functions in the human nervous system to activate muscles.

acidosis: Excessive acid in bodily fluids.

acne mechanica: Acne often triggered by heat or excess scrubbing or rubbing.

acne vulgaris: Common acne caused by inflammation of pores or hair follicles.

acupuncture: A Chinese science invented more than 1,000 years ago involving the insertion of very thin, sharp needles through the skin and into the underlying tissue to varying depths; intended to relieve pain, nausea, and so forth. The aim is to restore a harmonious balance between the yin and the yang energies of the life forces, or Chi.

acute pain: Pain that resolves itself quickly. *See also* **chronic pain**.

ADP: Adenosine diphosphate, the molecule that results from the removal of one phosphate from an ATP molecule by enzymes, releasing usable metabolic energy.

ATP: Adenosine triphosphate, the molecule that transports energy within the cells of the body.

adiposity: Fat; state of being fat.

adjuvants: Additives that allow needle-free administration of vaccines.

adult-onset diabetes: *See* **type 2 diabetes**.

aerobic: The stage in the metabolic generation of energy that uses oxygen to burn glucose.

aerobic capacity: The maximal ability of an individual's body to consume oxygen during physical activity.

aikido: Also known as "the way of the central spirit," a Japanese martial art that emphasizes nonresistance and the use of an opponent's momentum against him or her.

allergen: A substance that can cause an allergic reaction, such as a food or medicine.

allicin: A potent antioxidant.

alpha-linoleic acid: A type of omega-3 fatty acid.

alternative medicine: Practices used in place of standard conventional treatments.

Alzheimer's disease: A progressive brain disease that is the most common cause of dementia; formerly called presenile dementia.

amyloid beta plaques: Abnormal protein deposits found in the brains of Alzheimer's disease sufferers.

anabolic reactions: Reactions that consume energy and are used to resynthesize compounds.

anaerobic exercise: Fast-burst, high-intensity exercise used to build strength and muscle mass.

anaphylactic shock: A life-threatening condition with sudden onset; often brought on by severe allergic reaction.

andropause: Male menopause.

angina: Chest pain of cardiac origin caused by lack of blood flow.

angiogenesis: The in-growth of new blood vessels.

angioplasty: A medical procedure performed to widen existing coronary arteries.

anthocyanins: Powerful antioxidants.

antigravity training: Forms of exercise, such as swimming, that minimize the effects of the body's weight during a workout.

antioxidants: Substances that may protect cells by neutralizing the free radicals that damage cells and tissue.

apoptosis: Programmed cell death.

apple-shaped body: A body shape with more weight around the waist than around the hips.

arachidonic acid: A type of omega-6 fatty acid.

arrhythmias: Rhythm disturbances in the heart.

artificial menopause: Menopause brought on secondarily by removal of the ovaries for a medical reason; artificial menopause can also occur after radiation to the pelvis or chemotherapy for cancer and with some medications. This condition is usually abrupt and can lead to severe symptoms that may be treated with hormone replacement therapy.

asanas: Positions in yoga.

asthma: An inflammation of the small bronchial tubes at the very end of the airways into the tiny, sac-like alveoli; it leads to an inability to breathe air out.

atherosclerosis: Hardening of the arteries.

axon: A nerve fiber that carries electrical impulses.

axonal or dendritic pruning: Elimination of excess axonal branches and synaptic contacts often formed during early development.

ballistic stretching: A form of stretching that involves a bouncing motion; not beneficial for the body.

bariatric surgery: Weight-loss surgery performed on the obese that modifies the gastrointestinal tract.

basal metabolic rate: The speed at which the body burns energy while at rest.

bioavailability: The amount of a nutrient that the body can absorb and utilize.

biodegradable polymer technologies: A way to deliver booster doses of a vaccine long after an initial single injection.

bioidentical hormones: Hormone replacements made from natural, plant-based sources.

bisphosphonates: A family of drugs used to treat osteoporosis.

blue-zone communities: Areas of the world where the inhabitants tend to live longer and healthier lives.

board certification: Official recognition conferred on physicians who have met high standards of training and performance and have successfully passed rigid examinations in their areas of specialty.

board eligibility: Recognition conferred on physicians who have completed all requirements for certification except the examinations.

body mass index (BMI): The standard method of determining an individual's healthy weight range by height-to-weight ratio. To calculate, multiply your weight in pounds by 703, and divide by your height in inches squared. A BMI of less than 24.9 is considered normal weight; between 25 and 29.9 is overweight; and greater than 30 is obese. You can find a useful BMI calculator at http://www.cdc.gov.

bokken: Wooden training sword used in aikido.

brain-derived neurotrophic factor: A molecule involved in maintaining normal cognitive and emotional functioning.

BRCA: Tumor-suppressor gene mutations strongly linked to both breast and ovarian cancers.

bursa: Fluid-filled sacs that provide smooth, frictionless movement at or near a joint.

bursitis: Inflammation of the bursa.

calcification: Deposits of calcium salts in tissue, causing hardening.

calcitonin: A hormone produced by the thyroid gland that interferes with the osteoclasts and slows bone loss.

calisthenics: A system of body exercises; the term is a combination of words meaning "beauty" and "strength."

capillary network: Tiny vessels where the exchange of glucose, oxygen, and waste takes place.

carcinogen: Cancer-causing agent.

cardiorespiratory capacity: Ability of the heart and respiratory system to work together to generate energy.

CAT scan: Computerized axial tomography, a procedure used to identify disease or other abnormalities; a CAT scan machine uses computer technology to generate a three-dimensional image, or cross-section, of the body.

catabolic reactions: Metabolic reactions that break down molecules.

cellular distress: Stress on individual cells of the musculoskeletal system, arising from lack of oxygen, lack of glucose, or actual physical stress.

central obesity: A condition characterized by belly fat.

cholinesterase: An enzyme found primarily at nerve endings that helps transform acetylcholine into acetic acid and choline.

cholinesterase inhibitors: Drugs used to treat the symptoms of Alzheimer's disease.

chondroitin sulfate: A substance that prevents the breakdown of joint cartilage.

chronic obstructive pulmonary disease (COPD): A condition that includes the lung diseases chronic bronchitis and emphysema.

chronic pain: Pain that lasts a long time. *See also* **acute pain**.

circadian rhythm: The body's approximately 24-hour cycle of waking and sleeping; closely linked to the basic metabolism of cells and organs.

cirrhosis: Liver scarring, often the result of alcoholism.

clinical impression: A diagnosis professionals provide after a patient assessment.

cognition: Mental processes that include attention or focus; the acquisition of new information; memory; language and speech; and the translation of intention into movement through motor skills.

collagen protein: Proteins found in connective tissue and bones.

colonoscopy: A procedure using a flexible instrument to see inside the colon and rectum.

complementary medicine: The system of combining alternative treatments with conventional medicine.

complete protein: A protein source that has all the essential amino acids.

complex polysaccharide: A string of chemical sugars combined to form a starch.

concentric contraction: Muscle contraction in which the muscles shorten to produce motion against a force. This is a muscle's preferred way to work. *See also* **eccentric contraction**.

confounder: An extraneous variable in a medical study that might affect and threaten the validity of inferences and results of the study.

congestive heart failure: A form of cardiovascular disease in which structural or functional problems impair the heart's ability to provide adequate blood flow to the rest of the body.

conventional medicine: The system of medicine most often practiced by physicians and other health-care professionals, such as therapists, psychologists, pharmacists, and nurses.

conversational jog: Level of exertion at which an individual can carry on a conversation with a partner while running.

coronary artery disease: A condition in which plaque builds up inside the arteries of the heart.

cosmetic rhinoplasty: Surgical reshaping of the nose for cosmetic reasons.

cosmetic surgery: Surgical procedures performed to improve appearance.

cross-training: Engaging in a number of exercises for well-rounded aerobic and muscular development.

delayed-onset muscle soreness: A feeling of muscle pain a day or two after exercising.

dementia: Not a single specific disease but rather a condition that involves a progressive, chronic decline in cognitive function.

destructive exogenous free radicals: Free radicals that arise from outside sources, such as ultraviolet and other forms radiation, toxins, and pollutants.

DEXA scan: Dual-energy X-ray absorptiometry, a procedure that measures bone mineral density.

DASH diet: Dietary Approaches to Stop Hypertension, a way of eating designed to lower blood pressure developed by the American Heart Association.

diphenhydramine: An antihistamine; drowsiness may be a side effect.

disaccharide: A combination of two monosaccharides.

disuse atrophy: A degeneration of muscle mass due to inactivity.

docosahexaenoic acid: A type of omega-3 fatty acid.

dojo: Training arena for martial arts.

dynamic stretching: Stretching that uses speed, momentum, and active effort to exercise the muscle. *See also* **static stretching**.

eccentric contraction: An elongation of the muscle in response to a force—a "negative" motion. *See also* **concentric contraction**.

eicosapentaenoic acid (EPA): A type of omega-3 fatty acid.

elastic resistance bands: An exercise tool used in resistance training; the more the band is stretched, the greater the resistance.

eluting stent: A stent that releases anticlotting chemicals over time.

emotionally labile: Changeable, unpredictable.

endemic: An abnormality exhibiting high levels in an otherwise apparently healthy population.

endometrium: The lining of the uterus.

endorphins: Chemicals released by the brain that are similar in structure to the morphine or opium group of drugs.

enteric-coated aspirin: Aspirin treated with a special coating to pass through the stomach unaltered and to dissolve in the intestines, thus preventing stomach upsets.

epigallocatechin gallate: A highly powerful antioxidant found in tea.

erectile dysfunction: Chronic and consistent inability to reach and sustain an erection, along with the inability to engage in normal sexual activity.

estrogen: A female hormone produced by the body (especially in the ovaries) and necessary for the normal sexual development of the female.

estrogen decline: The decreased ovarian production and excretion of estrogen.

estrogen receptors: Molecules on the surface of certain cells in the body to which estrogen will bind.

executive function: A higher-level cognitive ability that guides complex behaviors, such as planning, decision making, and self-monitoring.

fascia: A layer of tissue that holds muscles together and provides a place for blood vessels, nerves, and interstitial or intercellular fluid to move.

fiber: The indigestible part of plant food (roughage) that creates bulk in the digestive system. It absorbs water, promotes defecation, and may aid in eliminating toxic wastes.

first-class lever: A lever with its fulcrum (support) between the point of resistance and the point of effort. An example in the human body is the motion used when the head is raised off the chest.

firsthand smoke: Smoke inhaled directly during the act of smoking a cigarette.

food allergies: Unexpected, unintended reactions to various foods or substances in foods.

forkhead box family: The *FOX* gene family, which produces transcription factors that play an important role in development and longevity.

FOXO: A subgroup of the *FOX* gene family that regulates metabolism and, possibly, lifespan.

FOXO3A: A gene variation that appears to have a powerful positive effect on life expectancy.

free graft: A graft that involves separating a very thin layer of skin from one part of the body and attaching it to another site.

free-motion machines: Exercise machines that help activate a number of muscles, rather than focusing on a narrow group.

free radicals: Very unstable and highly reactive atoms or groups of atoms with an odd (unpaired) number of electrons, which increases their tendency to bond with other molecules. Free radicals can damage cells and are believed to be responsible for aging, tissue damage, and possibly some diseases.

free weights: Equipment used in strength training to target specific muscle groups.

gamma wave: A brain wave pattern with a high frequency, thought to signify a high state of focus and concentration.

giant sets: A fitness routine in which a number of exercises are performed for the same muscle group with almost no rest between sets.

glucosamine: A substance that helps in the formation and repair of cartilage and other body tissues.

glucose: A simple sugar (monosaccharide) that is an important carbohydrate and the major energy source for the body.

glucose tolerance test: A test that measures the body's ability to use sugar (glucose), our main source of energy.

glycemic index: A numerical index that ranks carbohydrates (on a scale of 0 to 100) based on the rate of conversion of the carbohydrate to glucose inside the body and its entrance into the bloodstream.

glycogen: Glucose that can be stored in the liver and muscles for future use.

grading: A measure of the biologic aggressiveness of a cancer.

gross brain atrophy: Loss of neurons and their connections in the brain.

gynecomastia: Enlargement of the male breasts.

hakama: Long dress worn by kendo practitioners.

half-moon pose: A pose in yoga that strengthens the ankles and thighs and improves balance.

herbal supplements: Supplements derived from plants.

herniated lumbar discs: Ruptured or slipped discs in the spine.

HDL: High-density lipoprotein, or "good cholesterol," which removes excess cholesterol from the arteries and carries it to the liver for destruction. High levels of HDL are associated with decreased risk of heart disease.

HEPA filters: High-efficiency particulate air filters that can trap large numbers of small airborne particles and thus purify the air.

high-fructose corn syrup: A common sweetener composed of fructose and glucose.

high-intensity interval training: A form of training that involves short intervals of maximum-intensity exercise.

histamine: A substance released by the body during an allergic reaction.

homeopathy: A therapeutic method designed to treat disease by giving a patient minute doses of highly diluted, symptom-causing substances in an effort to stimulate the body's ability to heal itself. Little evidence exists to support the effectiveness of homeopathic treatment.

hormone manipulation: Changing the levels of estrogen vis à vis androgenic hormones.

hot flashes: Episodic flushing and sweating.

hydrophobic molecules: Molecules that do not dissolve in water.

hypertension: High blood pressure.

hypertrophy: An increase in mass or girth. For example, exercise can cause hypertrophy in muscle tissue.

hypervitaminosis: Excess vitamin intake.

inflammation: A bodily response to disease or tissue damage, resulting in swelling, redness, and pain.

insulin: An anabolic hormone in the pancreas responsible for moving glucose and other essential nutrients into cells.

insulin resistance: A condition in which normal levels of insulin are no longer sufficient to obtain the glucose-lowering effects of insulin in major tissues, such as fat, muscle, and liver.

insulin sensitivity: A condition in which very small amounts of insulin are required to keep the body's blood sugar levels in the normal range.

integrative (or **integrated**) **medicine**: A combination of conventional practices and proven alternative treatment options.

intercurrent disease: A new disease that intervenes during the course of another disease not related to the primary disease.

intermittent claudication: Pain caused by impeded blood flow to the legs, usually the calves.

intra-abdominal fat: Fat accumulating in and around the abdominal cavity and organs.

isometric contraction: A muscle exercise in which the muscle is not lengthened.

isotonic contraction: A muscle exercise in which the tension on the muscle stays the same despite a change in muscle length.

judo: From Japanese for "the gentle way," a sport derived from jujitsu that uses principles of balance and leverage.

jujitsu: A Japanese art of fighting without weapons, using holds, throws, and blows.

karate: The Japanese art of self-defense using kicks and punches.

kata: A technique of practicing the positions and movements of martial arts.

kendo: From the Japanese for "the way of the sword," the sport of fencing using a wooden or bamboo sword.

ketone bodies: Soluble compounds produced when fatty acids are broken down for energy in the body.

Krebs cycle: The energy-producing cycle in the body.

kung fu: A Chinese martial art that emphasizes not only fighting skills but also balance and concentration.

kyudo: Literally, "the way of the bow," the Japanese sport of archery, practiced for both physical and spiritual development.

laparoscopic surgery: Minimally invasive surgery using only a few small cuts in the body and an instrument through which interior structures can be seen.

ligaments: From the word "ligate," meaning "to bind or tie," ligaments connect bone to bone, not muscle to bone.

linoleic acid: A type of omega-6 fatty acid.

lipoproteins: Fat proteins.

LDL: low-density lipoprotein, fat protein that transports triglycerides from liver cells to fat cells, where they are stored; carries cholesterol in the blood and delivers it to cells throughout the body for tissue repair; and aids in the synthesis of vital chemicals, such as steroid hormones.

lutein: A carotenoid (organic pigment) associated with protection against age-associated macular degeneration.

lycopene: A carotenoid (organic pigment) found in high concentrations in the blood of healthy people; it is associated with protection against prostate cancer.

macronutrient: An essential nutrient required in relatively large amounts.

MRI: Magnetic resonance imaging, a detailed picture of the body's internal structure obtained without using X-rays.

mammoplasty: Surgical reshaping of the breast.

mantra: A word or phrase spoken repeatedly to relax the body and empty the mind.

martial arts: Arts of combat practiced as self-defense or as a sport or spiritual discipline.

maximum heart rate: A measure of anaerobic conditioning; calculated by subtracting one's age from 220.

meditation: A mental exercise designed to heighten concentration or spiritual awareness.

Mediterranean diet: A heart-healthy diet inspired by eating styles in Mediterranean countries that emphasize the consumption of healthy fats, fruits, vegetables, and fish with alcohol taken in moderation.

melanoma: A serious skin cancer.

melatonin: A sleep-regulating hormone also involved in modulating the circadian rhythms.

menopause: A phase in the life of a woman that begins 8–12 months after her menstrual periods have ceased.

menses: The menstrual cycle.

metabolic panel levels: Measures of certain compounds in the blood, such as blood sugar and electrolyte balances and calcium levels.

metabolic syndrome: A condition characterized by the presence of at least three of the following factors: abdominal or central obesity, high blood pressure, high triglycerides in the blood, low HDL cholesterol in the blood, and high blood glucose.

metabolism: All energy processes in the body, including consumption and expenditure of energy, as well as renewal of energy.

mindfulness: The awareness that arises through concentration and meditation.

minerals: Inorganic substances, such as calcium, magnesium, and potassium, required by the body in small amounts.

mitochondria: The cell's powerhouses and the source of energy in the engines of the cell.

mitochondrial enzymes: Biochemicals whose activities serve as markers of aging.

monosaccharides: Simple sugars, including glucose, galactose, and fructose.

monounsaturated fats: Fatty acids, considered heart healthy, that have only one double bond in the fatty acid chain; they are liquid at room temperature.

morbid obesity: A condition defined by being twice normal weight or 100 pounds overweight or having a BMI of more than 40.

morbidity: Nonlethal complications of a disease; rate of sickness.

mortality: Death; death rate.

motor neurons: Nerves that connect with muscle and stimulate muscle contraction.

motor unit: The combination of a single motor neuron, or nerve, and the muscles it activates.

multi-infarct dementia: Dementia caused by multiple small strokes in the brain, leading to damaged brain tissue.

myelin sheath: The protective membrane in the central nervous system.

natural menopause: The transition to total cessation of a woman's menstrual periods, which usually begins between 45 and 55 years of age and can take 5 to 10 years.

Nautilus exercise machine: A type of exercise training equipment.

neurofibrillary tangles: Buildup of proteins in the brains of Alzheimer's patients, resulting in cell death.

neuroimaging: Techniques to image the structure and functionality of the brain.

neuromuscular junction: A place in the body where the nerves meet the muscles; the point at which impulses are transmitted from the brain to the muscles.

neurons: Cells that serve as the building blocks of nervous tissue.

neuroplasticity: The brain's ability to reorganize and restructure itself by forming new neural connections.

obesity: State of excessive overweight; the third leading preventable cause of death in the United States, behind smoking and high blood pressure.

obstructive sleep apnea: A disorder in which a sleeping person's airway closes down; it causes chronic sleep deprivation and may result in serious health consequences.

omega-3 fatty acids: Highly unsaturated fats needed for the production of hormone-like compounds known as prostaglandins. A requirement for a healthy diet, they are found in coldwater fish, fish oils, and avocado.

omega-6 fatty acids: Unsaturated fats found in meat, corn oil, safflower oil, and sunflower oil; they tend to be overconsumed in the American diet and can increase inflammation, as in arthritis or in the arteries.

omenta: The apron of fat that protects internal organs.

organic: Biologic compounds or molecules found in nature that have a carbon base; may also refer to plant and animal products defined by a particular method of farming that uses no chemical pesticides and no chemical fertilizers.

osteoarthritis: Degeneration of cartilage.

osteoblasts: Cells that build up bone.

osteoclasts: Cells that break down bone and liberate calcium in the serum to compensate for low levels of calcium.

osteopenia: Low bone mass; characterized by a bone mineral density score of -1.0 to -2.5.

osteoporosis: A disorder characterized by weak and porous bones and a bone mineral density score of less than -2.5.

osteosarcoma: A serious form of bone cancer.

oxidation: A process whereby electrons are transferred from one molecule or atom to another, creating free radicals. Free radicals and oxidation reactions are a necessary part of normal host defenses, but excess oxidation reactions are damaging.

oxidative stress: The elevation of free radicals beyond the body's capability to neutralize them to safe levels. Excessive oxidative stress damages the cells and tissues, specifically the mitochondria.

palliation: Treatment of symptoms without the intent of curing the underlying disease.

parathyroid glands: Glands that produce parathyroid hormone, which stimulates the osteoclasts and controls the amount of calcium in the blood.

pear-shaped body: A body shape with more weight around the hips than around the waist.

pedicle graft: A graft in which a portion of the skin from the donor site remains attached to the donor area and the rest is attached to the recipient site, preserving the blood supply.

perimenopause: The beginning of irregularities in the menstrual cycle before the onset of menopause; also refers to the years leading up to menopause, which occurs between 8 and 12 months after the final menstrual period.

periodization: A way of dividing an exercise program into different sets that emphasize different training goals; also, a method for varying training at regular intervals.

periosteum: A covering on the bone.

Physicians' Health Study: A study designed to test the effects of aspirin and beta-carotene on cardiovascular disease and cancer.

phytoestrogens: Compounds developed from plants to mimic the effects of estrogen.

phytonutrients: Nutrient compounds that come from plants.

Pilates: An exercise system that emphasizes core strength, flexibility, and awareness of breathing.

platelet aggregation: A condition in which platelets gather in areas of inflammation or bleeding and cause clotting.

polyphenols: Common antioxidant molecules found in nature that may inhibit LDL oxidation and thereby prevent arterial plaque formation; found in red wine, grape juice, dark berries, and cherries.

polyunsaturated fats: Fatty acids that have two or more double bonds in the fatty acid chain; these fats are liquid at room temperature.

prefrontal cortex: The brain's planning center, located between the temples in the forehead and behind the eyes.

premature menopause: Early menopause brought on by various physical problems; common in women athletes, it may be related to different levels of male hormones. It also may be related to nutritional deficiencies, autoimmune diseases, and chronic stress.

probiotics: Active bacteria added to foods to promote digestive health; they can be found in yogurt. There is no evidence that these bacteria are any better than the bacteria already present in the colon.

prophylactic mastectomy: Preventive removal of the breast to protect against breast cancer.

prostate-specific antigen (PSA): An antigen used in screening for early, asymptomatic prostate cancer.

proteins: Complex substances made of amino acids whose main function is to build and repair tissue; proteins can be found in every tissue in the body.

psycho-oncology: A medical field that combines treatment of the psychological, emotional, and spiritual aspects of coping with a cancer diagnosis with the patient's physical care.

pyramids: A weight-training routine in which the weight is increased and the number of repetitions is decreased as one "climbs the pyramid"; the weight is then reduced and the repetitions are increased as one "descends the pyramid."

recommended daily allowance (RDA): The recommended daily dietary intake sufficient to meet the requirements of nearly all healthy individuals.

reconstructive surgery: Surgical procedure performed with the primary aim of improving function.

recovery time: The rest period after exercise that is essential to muscle and tissue repair and strength building.

relative risk: *See* **absolute risk.**

REM sleep: Rapid eye movement sleep, a period of sleep during which dreams occur; characterized by increased brain activity.

resistance training: Strength training that uses weights or other forms of resistance, such as elastic bands.

respirometer: An instrument for measuring the rate of respiration (exchange of oxygen and carbon dioxide).

resting pulse: The resting heart rate measured immediately after waking up in the morning and before getting out of bed.

resveratrol: An antioxidant polyphenol molecule produced by plants in response to their own stress; found in grape skins, grape juice, and red wine.

reverse osmosis purification system: Filtration method used for purifying water in which water is forced through a semipermeable membrane.

rhabdomyolysis: Breakdown of muscle tissue that releases myoglobin into the blood and thus can damage kidneys.

rheumatoid arthritis: Chronic joint inflammation that mainly attacks the joints in the hands and feet.

rickets: A calcium- and vitamin D–deficiency disease that damages bones.

RNA (ribonucleic acid): A type of molecule that plays a role in controlling the cell's chemical activities, including protein synthesis and transmission of genetic information.

satiety index: A system to measure the extent to which foods signal that you are full after eating.

saturated fats: Long carbon–fatty acid chains that have no double bond because the whole molecule is saturated with hydrogen ions. Saturated fats are solid at room temperature.

screening: A test for the presence of disease performed in the course of routine health care, regardless of whether the patient has symptoms or indications of illness.

sebum: The secretion from sebaceous (oil-producing) glands.

second-class lever: A lever that has its point of resistance (weight) between the fulcrum and the point of effort; the type used when a person stands on tiptoe.

secondhand smoke: Smoke that a smoker exhales and that another person breathes in after it has been diluted in the air.

selective estrogen receptor modulators: Synthetic molecules that can bind to estrogen receptors in the body and have estrogen-like effects on some parts of the body (e.g., bone) and antiestrogen effects in other areas (e.g., breast).

sepsis: A severe infection.

serum lipid profile: A blood test to determine risk of heart disease; measures levels of cholesterol, HDL, LDL, and triglycerides.

simple set: A certain number of repetitions of an exercise performed three times. For example, 10 bicep curls may be performed as one set.

sirtuins: Silent information regulator 2 (or SIR2) proteins, a group of molecules that regulates important biologic pathways, including metabolic processes and cell defenses, in many organisms, from bacteria up through more evolved organisms.

skeletal muscles: Striated muscles that enable movement and support the skeleton.

Slow Food Movement: A movement opposed to fast food that encourages local food traditions and less-intensive farming methods.

smooth muscles: Involuntary muscles found in the stomach, intestines, blood vessels, and bladder.

staging: A method of grouping cancer cases in categories based on the degree to which the cancer has spread.

standing bow-pulling pose: A yoga pose thought to increase circulation of the blood to the heart and lungs.

static stretching: Flexibility training in which the muscles are stretched while the body is at rest. *See also* **dynamic stretching**.

statin: A drug that blocks cholesterol production in the liver.

Glossary

stent: A prosthetic device designed to keep a widened artery open.

striated muscles: Voluntary muscles connected to bone that move parts of the skeleton; characterized by transverse stripes.

stroke volume: The amount of blood pumped out of the heart on each beat.

subperiosteal hematomas: Tiny hemorrhages under the covering of the bones, often caused by running.

sulfenic acid: A powerful antioxidant; a byproduct of the decomposition of allicin.

super sets: Exercise routines in which the individual alternates different kinds of exercises for the same muscle group.

superoxide radicals: Free radicals that tend to oxidize and provoke oxidative stress, damaging cells and tissues.

synapse: The point at which an impulse passes from one neuron to another.

synergy: A mutually advantageous situation in which the total result is greater than could be achieved by the individual elements.

synovial lining: The lining of the joint.

Tabata protocol: A workout that consists of 20 seconds of high-intensity exercise, such as sprinting, followed by 10 seconds of rest, repeated six or seven times.

tae kwon do: Korean art of self-defense characterized by kicks.

tai chi chuan (a.k.a. **tai chi**): A slow-motion, meditative exercise derived from Chinese martial arts.

tendinitis: Inflammation of a tendon.

tendon: Connective tissue that unites the muscle to the periosteum (covering of the bone). It is derived from the word *tendere*, "to stretch."

testosterone: The hormone produced in men's bodies that affects sexual features and development.

thimerosal: A mercury-containing preservative that was once used in vaccines.

third-class lever: A lever with its force application (point of effort) between the fulcrum and the resistance. An example would be the bent elbow in a weight-lifting exercise.

thirdhand smoke: The residue of tobacco products, including gases and particles, that remains in an environment after the airborne smoke has dissipated.

thrombolytic therapy: Use of drugs that can dissolve blood clots.

trans-fats: Unsaturated fats that have been hydrogenated so that they are more appropriate for baking and have increased shelf life.

transcription factor: A protein that controls the transfer of genetic information and plays an important role in cellular processes.

transient ischemic attacks (TIAs): Mini strokes.

triglycerides: Dietary fats composed of three fatty acids together with one molecule of glycerol. More than 90 percent of the fat in the body is in this form, as is most of the fat in food.

tryptophan: A precursor to melatonin, which is a sleep-regulating hormone; tryptophan is sometimes used to treat insomnia.

tumeric: A spice whose active component is curcumin, an antioxidant and anti-inflammatory.

tumor suppressor genes: Genes that help the body naturally fight off and prevent cancer.

type 1 diabetes: Sometimes called juvenile diabetes, an autoimmune disorder in which the individual does not produce any insulin because the beta cells do not function; patients must take insulin throughout their lives.

type 2 diabetes: Also called adult-onset diabetes, this is the more common form of diabetes, in which the body produces insulin but does not use it effectively. Diagnosed in those with a fasting blood sugar greater than 126 milligrams per deciliter or an oral glucose tolerance test greater than 200.

type I muscle fibers: Slow-twitch muscle fibers that use oxygen for energy and are extremely fatigue resistant. They are found, for example, in postural muscles.

type II muscle fibers: Fast-twitch muscle fibers characterized by quick contraction time. Type IIA fibers are fast oxidative fibers, which are less fatigue resistant and are typical of a sprinter's muscles. Type IIB fibers are fast glycolytic fibers that operate with the production of lactic acid instead of oxygen and carbon dioxide. They are used for explosive bursts of activity and fatigue easily.

unsaturated fats: Fats in which double bonds exist between the carbon molecules; they take the form of monounsaturated and polyunsaturated fats.

Valsalva maneuver: A technique of forcing air against a closed airway to test cardiac function.

vascular dementia: A common type of dementia caused by impaired blood flow to the brain. It may be brought on by a stroke, meaning that an artery is closed. It may also occur after a series of small strokes that block vessels.

venous thromboembolism: A condition in which blood clots migrate to the lung.

ventricular fibrillation: Rapid, erratic heartbeats that result in the ventricles' failure to pump blood; lethal arrhythmia.

visceral fat: Belly fat inside the abdomen.

visceral organs: The organs inside the abdomen and around the belly.

vitamer: One of two or more related chemical substances that fulfills the same specific vitamin function.

vitamins: Organic chemical compounds that the body must obtain from external sources because they cannot be manufactured internally.

VLDL: Very low-density lipoprotein. *See* **LDL**.

VO$_2$ max: An indicator of aerobic endurance—the maximum volume of oxygen (O$_2$) that an individual can use during exercise, measured in liters of oxygen per minute.

warrior pose: A yoga pose that strengthens the legs and opens the chest and shoulders.

weight training: The practice of lifting weights or pushing against resistance to build muscles.

yoga: A system of exercises, originating in India, designed to promote well-being of the body and mind.

zazen: Zen meditation.

Zen Buddhism: A school of Buddhism that focuses on meditation as the path to enlightenment.

Glossary

Bibliography

Note: Professor Goodman neither endorses nor necessarily agrees with all content in the websites listed in this bibliography. He lists them as starting places—resources that may have some valuable information or further links. In the world of medicine, information changes quickly; on the Internet, websites change quickly, as well. Be discriminating and discerning and use these sites to work for you.

If a website is marked with an asterisk, some of its contents are free and no login is required, but if you sign up (and sometimes pay), you will receive newsletters, full access to archives, and other bonus materials.

General: Reading

Dorland's Illustrated Medical Dictionary with CD-ROM. 28th ed. Philadelphia, PA: Saunders, 2009.

Tortora, G. J., and B. H. Derrickson. *Principles of Anatomy and Physiology.* Hoboken, NJ: Wiley and Sons, 2008.

General: Internet Resources

*American Pain Foundation. http://www.painfoundation.org.

*Blue Zones. http://www.bluezones.com.

Centers for Disease Control and Prevention. http://www.cdc.gov.

Centers for Disease Control and Prevention, Vaccination Schedule. http://www.cdc.gov/vaccines/recs/schedules/adult-schedule.htm.

Center for Science in the Public Interest. http://www.cspinet.org.

*Consumer Reports. http://www.consumerreports.org.

Informed Medical Decisions. http://www.informedmedicaldecisions.org.

*The Lancet. http://www.thelancet.com.

Mayo Clinic. http://www.mayoclinic.com.

Medline Plus. http://www.nlm.nih.gov/medlineplus.

The Merck Manual of Medical Information. http://www.merck.com/mmpe/index.html.

*The New England Journal of Medicine. http://content.nejm.org.

Physicians Committee for Responsible Medicine. http://www.pcrm.org.

Science-Based Medicine. http://www.sciencebasedmedicine.org.

Science Daily. http://www.sciencedaily.com/news/health_medicine.

*Scientific American. http://www.scientificamerican.com/health.

*UC Berkeley Wellness Letter. http://www.wellnessletter.com.

*Up to Date. http://www.uptodate.com.

*Web MD. http://www.webmd.com.

Yale Griffin Prevention Research Center. http://www.yalegriffinprc.org.

Aging: Reading

Bartecchi, Carl E., and Robert W. Schrier. *Living Healthier and Longer—What Works, What Doesn't.* Pueblo, CO: MFTP Publications, 2008. http://www.healthierlongerlife.org.

Buettner, Dan. *The Blue Zones: Lessons from the People Who've Lived the Longest.* Washington, DC: National Geographic Society, 2008.

Chen, Pauline W. *Final Exam: A Surgeon's Reflections on Mortality.* New York: Vintage Books, 2008.

Clark, Etta. *Growing Old Is Not for Sissies II: Portraits of Senior Athletes.* 1st ed. Petaluma, CA: Pomegranate Communications, 1995.

Dass, Ram. *Conscious Aging: On the Nature of Change and Facing Death.* Boulder, CO: Sounds True Recordings, 2006.

———. *Still Here Now: Embracing Aging, Changing and Dying.* New York: Riverhead Trade, 2001.

Frankl, Viktor E. *Man's Search for Meaning.* Boston: Beacon Press, 2006.

Hayflick, Leonard. *How and Why We Age*. New York: Ballantine Books, 1994.

Kubler-Ross, Elisabeth. *On Death and Dying*. New York: Scribner, 1997.

Langer, Ellen J. *Counterclockwise: Mindful Health and the Power of Possibility*. New York: Ballantine Books, 2009.

Lawrence-Lightfoot, Sara. *The Third Chapter: Passion, Risk, and Adventure in the 25 Years after 50*. New York: Farrar, Strauss, and Giroux, 2009.

Moyers, Bill. *On Our Own Terms* (PBS DVD series; available at http://www.pbs.org/wnet/onourownterms). Films for the Humanities and Sciences. Aired September 10–13, 2000. PBS: 2000.

Olshansky, S. Jay, and Bruce A. Carnes. *The Quest for Immortality: Science at the Frontiers of Aging*. New York: W.W. Norton, 2001.

————. "A Position Statement on Human Aging." *Journals of Gerontology A: Biological Sciences and Medical Sciences* 75 (2002): 292–97.

Rowe, John W. and Robert L. Kahn. *Successful Aging*. New York: Dell, 1999.

Rudman, Daniel. "Effects of Human Growth Hormone in Men Over 60 Years Old." *New England Journal of Medicine* 323 (July 5, 1990). Available at http://content.nejm.org/content/vol323/issue1/index.dtl.

Sagan, Carl, and Ann Druyan. *The Demon-Haunted World: Science as a Candle in the Dark*. New York: Ballantine Books, 1997.

Saunders, Cicely, Mary Baines, and Robert Dunlop. *Living with Dying: A Guide to Palliative Care*, 3rd ed. Oxford, England: Oxford University Press, 1995.

Schachter-Shalomi, Zalman. *From Age-ing to Sage-ing: A Profound New Vision of Growing Older*. New York: Grand Central Publishing, 1997.

Valliant, George. *Aging Well: Surprising Guideposts to a Happier Life from the Landmark Harvard Study of Adult Development*. New York: Little, Brown and Company, 2003.

————. *Adaptation to Life*. Boston: Little, Brown, 1977.

————. *Spiritual Evolution: How We Are Wired for Faith, Hope, and Love.* New York: Broadway Press, 2008.

Weil, Andrew. *Healthy Aging: A Lifelong Guide to Your Well-Being.* New York: Anchor Books, 2005.

Aging: Internet Resources

Alliance for Aging Research. http://www.agingresearch.org/section/directory.

Healthy Aging. http://www.nia.nih.gov/HealthInformation.

Healthy at 100. http://www.healthyat100.org.

"Believed to Be World's Oldest, Woman in France Dies at 122." *Supercentenarian.com.* http://www.supercentenarian.com/oldest/jeanne-calment.html.

*National Council on Aging. http://www.ncoa.org.

National Institute on Aging. http://www.nia.nih.gov.

NIHSeniorHealth. http://www.nihseniorhealth.gov.

Stanford Aging Clinical Research Center. http://www.stanford.edu/~yesavage/ACRC.html.

Death and Dying: Internet Resources

Compassion and Choices: Choice and Care at the End of Life. http://www.compassionandchoices.org.

Hospicenet.org. http://www.hospicenet.org.

"End of Life Issues." *Medline Plus.* http://www.nlm.nih.gov/medlineplus/endoflifeissues.html.

On Our Own Terms: Moyers on Dying. http://www.pbs.org/wnet/onourownterms/index.html.

General Nutrition: Reading

Arenson, Gloria. *A Substance Called Food: How to Understand, Control and Recover from Addictive Eating.* New York: McGraw-Hill, 1989.

———. *Desserts Is Stressed Spelled Backwards: Overcoming and Controlling Compulsive Eating and Bulimia.* Santa Barbara, CA: Brockart Books, 2009.

Chopra, Deepak. *Perfect Health: The Complete Mind-Body Guide.* Rev. ed. New York: Harmony, 2001.

David, Marc. *The Slow Down Diet: Eating for Pleasure, Energy, and Weight Loss.* Rochester, VT: Healing Arts Press, 2005.

Gifford, K. Dun, and Sara Baer-Sinnott. *The Oldways Table: Essays and Recipes from the Culinary Think Tank.* Berkeley, CA: Ten Speed Press, 2007.

Hyman, Mark and Mark Liponis. *Ultraprevention: The 6-Week Plan That Will Make You Healthy for Life.* New York: Atria, 2005.

Jacobs, David and Linda Tabsell. "Food, Not Nutrients, Is the Fundamental Unit in Nutrition." *Nutrition Reviews* 65 (October 2007: 439–50).

Kessler, David A. *The End of Overeating: Taking Control of the Insatiable American Appetite.* New York: Rodale Books, 2009.

Kingsolver, Barbara, Camille Kingsolver, and Steven L. Hopp. *Animal, Vegetable, Miracle: A Year of Food Life.* New York: Harper-Perennial, 2007.

Lappe, Francis Moore, and Anna Lappe. *Hope's Edge: The Next Diet for a Small Planet.* New York: Tarcher, 2003.

Nestle, Marion. *What to Eat.* San Francisco: North Point Press, 2007.

———. *Food Politics: How the Food Industry Influences Nutrition and Health.* Rev. ed. California Studies in Food and Culture. Berkeley, CA: University of California Press, 2007.

Pollan, Michael. *The Omnivore's Dilemma: A Natural History of Four Meals.* New York: Penguin, 2007.

———. *In Defense of Food: An Eater's Manifesto*. New York: Penguin, 2008.

Robbins, John. *Healthy at 100: The Scientifically Proven Secrets of the World's Healthiest and Longest-Lived Peoples*. New York: Ballantine Books, 2007.

Robbins, John and Dean Ornish. *The Food Revolution: How Your Diet Can Help Save Your Life and Our World*. San Francisco: Conari Press, 2001.

Roizen, Michael F. and Mehmet C. Oz. *You Staying Young: The Owner's Manual for Extending Your Warranty*. New York: Free Press, 2007.

Spain, T., and L. Spain. *Fat: What No One Is Telling You* (PBS DVD; available at http://www.shoppbs.org). Twin Cities Public Television, Inc., 2007.

Taubes, Gary. *Good Calories, Bad Calories: Fats, Carbs and the Controversial Science of Diet and Health*. New York: Vintage, 2008.

General Nutrition: Internet Resources

American Diabetes Association. http://www.diabetes.org.

American Dietetic Association. http://www.eatright.org/cps/rde/xchg/ada/hs.xsl/nutrition.html.

The American Journal of Clinical Nutrition. http://www.ajcn.org.

Cornell University Food and Brand Lab. http://www.foodpsychology.cornell.edu.

The DASH Diet Eating Plan. http://www.dashdiet.org.

Food and Behaviour Research. http://www.fabresearch.org.

The Food Revolution. http://www.foodrevolution.org.

Glycemic Index and GI Database. http://www.glycemicindex.com.

International Association for the Study of Obesity. http://www.iaso.org/index.asp.

Mediterranean Foods Alliance. http://www.mediterraneanmark.org.

National Institutes of Health Office of Dietary Supplements. http://ods.od.nih.gov.

*Oldways. http://www.oldwayspt.org.

MyPyramid.gov. http://www.mypyramid.gov/index.html.

U.S. Food and Drug Administration. http://www.fda.gov.

World's Healthiest Foods. http://www.whfoods.com.

Zorba Paster on Your Health. http://www.wpr.org/Zorba.

Nutrition for Children and Youth: Reading

American Dietetic Association. "Dietary Guidance for Healthy Children Aged 2–11 Years. Position of the ADA." *Journal of the American Dietetic Association* 99 (1999): 93–101.

Nutrition for Children and Youth: Internet Resources

*Farm to School. http://www.farmtoschool.org.

"Resources." *The s'Cool Food Initiative.* http://www.scoolfood.org/resources/resources.cfm.

"Role of Nutrition in Learning and Behavior: A Resource List for Professionals." *U.S. Department of Agriculture Food and Nutrition Information Center.* http://www.nal.usda.gov/fnic/service/learning.pdf.

"MyPyramid for Preschoolers." *MyPyramid.gov.* http://www.mypyramid.gov/preschoolers/index.html.

*"Local Wellness Policy." *USDA Food and Nutrition Service: Team Nutrition.* http://www.fns.usda.gov/tn/healthy/wellnesspolicy.html.

*"Nutrition Diet and Weight Issues among Children and Adolescents—How Many Children And Teens Are Overweight?, Why Are So Many Children And Teens Overweight?, Health Risks And Consequences." *LibraryIndex. com.* http://www.libraryindex.com/pages/110/Diet-Nutrition-Weight-Issues-among-Children-Adolescents.html.

Cookbooks

Bittman, Mark. *How to Cook Everything: 2,000 Simple Recipes for Great Food.* Hoboken, NJ: Wiley Books, 2008.

————. *Food Matters: A Guide to Conscious Eating with More than 75 Recipes.* New York: Simon & Schuster, 2008.

Dayuff, Roberta Larson. *American Dietetic Association Complete Food and Nutrition Guide.* Hoboken, NJ: Wiley, 2006.

Feuer, Janice. *Fruit-Sweet and Sugar-Free: Prize-Winning Pies, Cakes, Pastries, Muffins and Breads from the Ranch Kitchen Bakery.* Rochester, VT: Healing Arts Press, 1992.

Mateljan, George. *The World's Healthiest Foods: Essential Guide for the Healthiest Way of Eating.* Seattle, WA: World's Healthiest Foods, 2006.

Gardening, Farming, Local Produce: Reading

Bartholomew, Mel. *All New Square Foot Gardening: Grow More in Less Space!* Franklin, TN: Cool Springs Press, 2006.

Gardening, Farming, Local Produce: Internet Resources

*Buy Local. http://www.buylocalfood.com.

*Community Alliance with Family Farmers. http://www.caff.org.

*The Daily Green. http://www.thedailygreen.com.

Eat Well Guide. http://www.eatwellguide.org.

Eat Wild. http://www.eatwild.com.

Eat Your Roots. http://www.eatyourroots.org/Home_Page.html.

Food Routes. http://www.foodroutes.org.

Healthy Eating Politics. http://www.healthy-eating-politics.com/index.html.

*Institute for Food and Development Policy. http://www.foodfirst.org.

*Kitchen Gardeners International. http://www.kitchengardeners.org.

Local Harvest. http://www.localharvest.org.

Natural News. http://www.naturalnews.com.

The Organic Center. http://organic.insightd.net.

Seafood Choices Alliance, http://www.seafoodchoices.com.

Seafood Watch Program, http://www.seafoodwatch.org.

USDA Agricultural Marketing Service Farmers Market Search. http://apps. ams.usda.gov/FarmersMarkets.

Exercise

Goldstein, Mel, and David Tanner. *Swimming Past 50*. Champaign, IL: Human Kinetics, 1999.

Hartmann, Thom. *Walking Your Blues Away: How to Heal the Mind and Create Emotional Well-Being*. Rochester, NY: Park Street Press, 2006.

Exercise: Internet Resources

About.com: Yoga. http://yoga.about.com.

American College of Sports Medicine. http://www.acsm.org.

Exercise Is Medicine. http://www.exerciseismedicine.org.

Mayo Clinic Staff. *Video: Yoga for Stress Management*. http://www. mayoclinic.com/health/yoga/MM00650.

MSN Health & Fitness, Diet & Fitness. http://health.msn.com/nutrition.

MyStart!   Online.   http://www.americanheart.org/presenter. jhtml?identifier=3053103.

National Safety Foundation. http://www.nsf.org.

Racewalk.com. http://www.racewalk.com/HowTo/Introduction.asp.

Tabata Protocol. http://www.tabataprotocol.com.

The Walking Site. http://www.thewalkingsite.com.

Yoga Health Foundation. http://www.yogahealthfoundation.org/index.php.

Yoga Journal. http://www.yogajournal.com.

Women's Health: Reading

Brizendine, Louann. *The Female Brain.* New York: Broadway Books, 2006.

Northrup, Christiane *The Wisdom of Menopause: Creating Physical and Emotional Health and Healing During the Change.* New York: Bantam Books, 2006.

————. *Women's Bodies, Women's Wisdom: Creating Physical and Emotional Health and Healing.* New York: Bantam Books, 2006.

Women's Health: Internet Resources

North American Menopause Society. http://www.menopause.org/Consumers. aspx.

WomensHealth.gov. http://www.womenshealth.gov.

Women's Health Initiative. http://www.whi.org.

Men's Health: Reading

Crowley, Chris, and Henry Lodge. *Younger Next Year: Live Strong, Fit and Sexy until You're 80 and Beyond.* New York: Workman Publishing, 2007.

Men's Health: Internet Resources

"Men's Health." *Medline Plus.* http://www.nlm.nih.gov/medlineplus/ menshealth.html.

Children's and Adolescents' Health: Internet Resources

"Attention-Defecit/Hyperactivity Disorder (ADHD)." *Centers for Disease Control and Prevention.* http://www.cdc.gov/ncbddd/adhd/index.html.

"Advisory Committee on Immunization Practices." *Centers for Disease Control and Prevention.* http://www.cdc.gov/vaccines/recs/ACIP/default. htm.

Juvenile Diabetes Research Foundation. http://www.jdrf.org.

*No Child Left Inside. http://www.cbf.org/Page.aspx?pid=687.

Mental Health: Reading

Combs, Deidre. *Worst Enemy, Best Teacher: How to Survive and Thrive with Opponents, Competitors, and the People Who Drive You Crazy.* Novato, CA: New World Library, 2005.

Honore, Carl. *In Praise of Slowness: Challenging the Cult of Speed.* New York: Harper, 2004.

Kabat-Zinn, Jon. *Full Catastrophe Living: Using the Wisdom of Your Body and Mind to Face Stress, Pain, and Illness.* New York: Delta, 1990.

————. *Mindfulness for Beginners.* Louisville, CO: Sounds True Recordings, 2006.

Lyubomirsky, Sonja. *The How of Happiness: A New Approach to Getting the Life You Want.* New York: Penguin, 2008.

Siegel, Daniel J. *The Mindful Brain: Reflection and Attunement in the Cultivation of Well-Being.* New York: W.W. Norton, 2007.

Mental Health: Internet Resources

*Center for Mindfulness in Medicine, Healthcare and Society. http://www. umassmed.edu/content.aspx?id=41252.

*"Stress Reduction Program." Center for Mindfulness in Medicine, Healthcare and Society. http://www.umassmed.edu/Content.aspx?id=41254 &LinkIdentifier=id.

Mayo Clinic Staff. "Relaxation Techniques: Learn Ways to Reduce Your Stress." http://www.mayoclinic.com/health/relaxation-technique/sr00007.

Sleep: Internet Resources

American Academy of Sleep Medicine. http://www.aasmnet.org/PatientsPublic.aspx.

American Academy of Sleep Medicine. *Sleepcenters.org.* http://www.sleepcenters.org.

————. *Sleepeducation.com.* http://www.sleepeducation.com/.

Caregiving: Internet Resources

Lots of Helping Hands. http://www.lotsahelpinghands.com.

National Center on Caregiving. http://www.caregiver.org.

National Family Caregivers Association. http://www.nfcacares.org.

Healthy Choices: Reading

Combs, Deidre. *Worst Enemy, Best Teacher: How to Survive and Thrive with Opponents, Competitors, and the People Who Drive You Crazy.* Novato, CA: New World Library, 2005 .

Cousins, Norman. *Anatomy of an Illness as Perceived by the Patient.* New York: W.W. Norton, 1979.

Goleman, Daniel. *Ecological Intelligence: How Knowing the Hidden Impacts of What We Buy Can Change Everything.* New York: Broadway Business, 2009.

Lynn, Joanne. *Sick to Death and Not Going to Take It Anymore! Reforming Health Care for the Last Years of Life.* Berkeley, CA: University of California Press, 2004.

Singh, Simon, and Ernst Edzard. *Trick or Treatment: Undeniable Facts about Alternative Medicine.* New York: W.W. Norton, 2008.

Snyderman, Nancy L. *Medical Myths That Can Kill You and the 101 Truths That Will Save, Extend and Improve Your Life.* New York: Three Rivers Press, 2008.

Healthy Choices: Internet Resources

Centers for Disease Control and Prevention. *Adult Immunization Schedule.* http://www.cdc.gov/vaccines/recs/schedules/adult-schedule.htm.

Environmental Working Group. http://www.ewg.org.

Memorial Sloan-Kettering Cancer Center. *About Herbal Medicine.* http://www.mskcc.org/mskcc/html/11570.cfm.

National Center for Complementary and Alternative Medicine. http://nccam.nih.gov.

National Center for Complementary and Alternative Medicine. *Time to Talk.* nccam.nih.gov/timetotalk.

*Preventive Medicine Research Institute. http://www.pmri.org/research.html.

U.S. Department of Health and Human Services. *Household Products Database.* http://householdproducts.nlm.nih.gov/index.htm.

U.S. Environmental Protection Agency. *Safewater.* http://www.epa.gov/safewater/dwh/index.html.

————. *Safewater Consumer Confidence Reports.* http://www.epa.gov/safewater/ccr/index.html.

Medical Associations: Internet Resources

*American Academy of Family Physicians. http://www.aafp.org.

*American Academy of Pediatrics. http://www.aap.org.

American Board of Medical Specialties. http://www.abms.org/.

*American Cancer Society. http://www.cancer.org.

*American College of Obstetricians and Gynecologists. http://www.acog.org.

*American College of Physicians. http://www.acponline.org.

*American College of Surgeons. http://www.facs.org.

American Society of Anesthesiologists. http://www.asahq.org.

American Society of Clinical Oncology. http://www.asco.org.

National Cancer Institute. http://www.cancer.gov.

Society of General Internal Medicine. http://www.sgim.org.

State Boards of Medicine. http://www.ama-assn.org/ama/pub/category/2645. html.

U.S. Department of Health and Human Services. Hospital Compare, http://www.hospitalcompare.hhs.gov.

U.S. Department of Veterans Affairs: Veterans Health. http://www. myhealth.va.gov.

Selected Studies

Fiatarone M. A., E. F. O'Neill, N. Doyle, K. M. Clements, S. B. Roberts, J. J. Kehayias, L. A. Lipsitz, and W. J. Evans. "The Boston FICSIT Study: The Effects of Resistance Training and Nutritional Supplementation on Physical Frailty in the Oldest Old." *Journal of the American Geriatrics Society* 41 (March 1993): 333–37.

Harvard Study of Adult Development, http://adultdev.bwh.harvard. edu/research-SAD.html. See in Aging section: "Aging Well: Surprising Guideposts to a Happier Life from the Landmark Harvard Study of Adult Development" by George Valliant.

Nurses' Health Study, http://www.channing.harvard.edu/nhs/ and http:// www.brighamandwomens.org/publicaffairs/NursesHealthStudy.aspx.

Women's Health Initiative, http://www.nhlbi.nih.gov/whi/index.html.

Notes

Notes

Notes

Notes

Notes

Notes

Notes

Notes